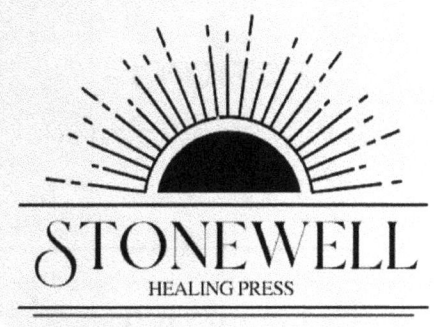

© Stonewell Healing Press, 2025
 All rights reserved.
This book is a labor of care. Please do not copy, share, or distribute any part of it—digitally or physically—without written permission from the author or publisher, except for brief excerpts used in reviews or critical articles. Your respect helps this work reach others who need it.
This workbook is not a replacement for therapy, crisis support, or mental health treatment. It's meant to offer reflection, comfort, and growth—not clinical care. If you're struggling, please reach out to a licensed professional. You matter too much to go through it alone.
Every effort has been made to ensure this content is accurate, responsible, and thoughtful. The author and publisher cannot guarantee outcomes and are not liable for misuse or misinterpretation of the material.

Thank you for being here. We're honored to walk beside you.

M. Tourangeau
Stonewell Healing Press

TABLE OF CONTENTS

SECTION 1 -   12
Why Birth Trauma Hurts So Much

SECTION 2-   40
The Moment Everything Changed

SECTION 3 -   66
When My Body Wasn't Safe Anymore

SECTION 4 -   84
The Aftershock – When Everyone Moved On but I Couldn't

SECTION 5-   110
Touch, Sex, and Sensitivity – When Intimacy Feels Impossible

SECTION 6   136
What Happened to Me? Making Sense of the Medical Mayhem

Stonewell Healing Press

TABLE OF CONTENTS

SECTION 7 -   **158**

Invisible Grief – Mourning What Wasn't Supposed to Be Lost

SECTION 8-   **176**

Loving While Still Hurting – Parenting When Bonding Is Hard

SECTION 9 -   **202**

If I Ever Do This Again – Fear, Decisions, and Autonomy After Trauma

---

SECTION 10 -   **234**

The Partner Gap – Feeling Alone in the Aftermath

SECTION 11 -   **270**

When Help Didn't Help – Medical Betrayal and Systemic Gaslighting

---

BONUS SECTION   **298**

Stonewell Healing Press

Dedicated to those who were left traumatized on what was meant to be the most beautiful day of their lives.

STONEWELL HEALING PRESS

HOW TO USE THIS WORKBOOK

Take your time with this. The more you pause to really think about each question and answer honestly, the more space you create for reflection. And with deeper reflection, this experience can open up new understanding and healing you might not expect.

Be honest with yourself—there's no judgment here. This is your private space. If you want, you can even throw this book away or burn it later to keep your secrets safe. That said, be mindful of how much you dive in. Healing and reflection around tough, sensitive topics can bring up strong feelings—and yes, it can get triggering. So here's your gentle trigger warning.

The real progress comes when you practice the skills, not just read about them. The more you try them out in your life, the more helpful this workbook will be.

STONEWELL HEALING PRESS

ASSESSMENT

WHERE AM I NOW?

Before we begin, take a moment to honestly check in with yourself by rating these statements on a scale from 1 (not at all) to 10 (completely):

1-10

1   I feel at home in my own body.

2   I can sit with my grief without shutting down.

3   I trust my choices about my body and health.

4   I can experience touch or intimacy without fear.

5   I can speak about my birth experience honestly.

6   I feel emotionally connected to myself and others.

7   I allow myself moments of joy without guilt.

8   I believe my feelings and experiences are valid.

SECTION ONE

Why Birth Trauma Hurts So Much

You might still be asking yourself: Was it really that bad? Shouldn't I just be grateful? Birth trauma is often minimized — by others, and even by ourselves. But here's the truth: when something meant to be sacred becomes terrifying, disempowering, or life-threatening, the imprint goes far deeper than the event itself. Birth trauma isn't about pain tolerance. It's about safety — and when safety shatters in a moment when your body was most vulnerable, your whole system remembers.

This chapter is your permission slip to name it: what happened matters. Not because you're weak. But because your body, your heart, and your nervous system were doing their best to survive something overwhelming. That survival response doesn't disappear just because the baby is here. This is your space to understand why you feel what you feel — and to start gently making sense of it, one breath at a time.

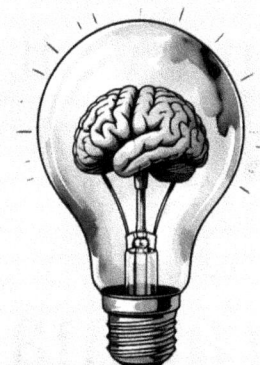

Making Sense Of It
The Lasting Weight of Birth Trauma

Birth is supposed to be a milestone, a moment of completion, a celebration. But when trauma intervenes—when fear, helplessness, or violation enters—something fundamental shifts. The body and mind are built to survive, and in those moments when safety is threatened, every system is on high alert. Your muscles tighten, your heart races, your breath shortens. Your brain flips into survival mode: the amygdala lights up, memory circuits encode threat with brutal precision, and the rational part of your mind, the prefrontal cortex, takes a backseat. This is your body doing its job, protecting you in a moment of extreme vulnerability—but it also means your nervous system remembers long after the hospital room is empty and the baby is home.

Psychologically, trauma after birth is complex because it touches multiple layers of identity. You may have expected control over your body, your birth plan, or your emotions—and when that control is stripped away, it can feel like a personal failing. But it's not failing—it's survival. The mismatch between what you expected and what actually happened creates cognitive dissonance, self-doubt, and sometimes shame. Socially, we live in a culture that glorifies birth while silencing discomfort. Phrases like "at least the baby is healthy" or "you should just be grateful" can unintentionally invalidate deep, real feelings. Friends, family, and even medical providers may minimize the experience, leaving trauma survivors isolated, questioning their own perceptions, and unsure if their feelings are "real" enough to matter.

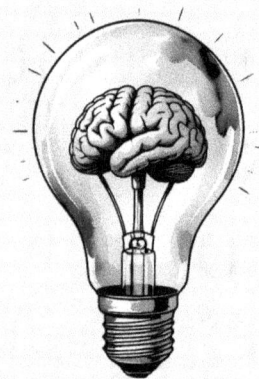

Making Sense Of It
The Lasting Weight of Birth Trauma

The imprint of birth trauma isn't just emotional—it's profoundly embodied. Some mothers describe feeling disconnected from their bodies, from their babies, or even from the joy they thought would accompany birth. Sleep disturbances, hypervigilance, flashbacks, or sudden anxiety can surface unpredictably, sometimes triggered by sights, sounds, or smells that echo the original experience. These reactions are not signs of weakness—they are the language of a body trying to reconcile what happened with what it expected.

On a deeper level, birth trauma touches identity, agency, and trust. You may question your strength, your choices, or your capacity to protect yourself and your child. Relationships can feel strained as you navigate your grief, your fear, or your sense of loss. Even moments meant for connection—like holding your newborn—can be tinged with disorientation, anger, or sadness. This isn't a reflection of your love or your maternal instincts; it's the aftershock of an experience that your mind and body are still working to integrate.

Understanding this truth—seeing your reactions as natural responses to violation of trust, control, or safety—is the first step toward reclaiming yourself. Healing begins when you allow yourself to acknowledge that your experience mattered, that your body and mind were doing what they needed to survive, and that your feelings are valid, even if they feel contradictory. It's not about forgetting the trauma or forcing yourself to "move on."

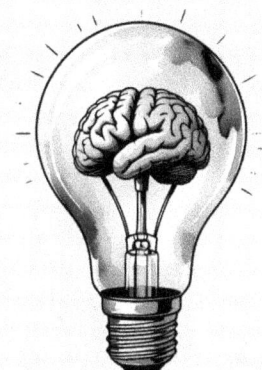

Making Sense Of It
The Lasting Weight of Birth Trauma

Every heartbeat, every breath, every tension in your body tells a story about survival. By learning to listen—to your nervous system, your emotions, and your thoughts—you can begin to untangle the aftermath of trauma from your sense of self. You can start to reclaim the trust in your body, the agency over your choices, and the emotional space to hold both your grief and your love. Birth trauma leaves a mark, but it does not define your strength, your resilience, or your capacity to heal. It simply asks for acknowledgment, compassion, and care—first from yourself, and then from the world around you.

What does the word "trauma" bring up in me right now?

You don't have to adopt this word if it doesn't feel right. But notice what happens in your body when you consider that your birth might have been traumatic. Do you tense? Do you feel relief? Fear?

What does the word "trauma" bring up in me right now?

In what moments did I feel like I disappeared, or no one was listening?

Trauma can often feel like invisibility — like screaming silently. Were there moments during or after the birth when you felt erased, silenced, or small? Write to those moments as if you're reclaiming your voice now.

In what moments did I feel like I disappeared, or no one was listening?

What part of me still doesn't believe I'm "allowed" to feel this way?

Is there an inner critic that tells you you're overreacting? A part of you afraid to be judged? Let that part speak. Then respond from a place of compassion: "I hear you. And I'm still allowed to hurt."

What part of me still doesn't believe I'm "allowed" to feel this way?

What have I tried to tell myself to make this seem less painful?

Many of us minimize our pain to cope. What mantras or phrases have you used — even if they don't feel true? ("It wasn't that bad." "At least the baby's healthy.") Gently examine what's underneath those thoughts.

What have I tried to tell myself to make this seem less painful?

Where in my body do I still feel the imprint of what happened?

Scan your body slowly. Is there tightness in your jaw? A flutter in your chest? A blankness in your stomach? This isn't about fixing — just noticing. Your body might be carrying the story more clearly than your mind.

Where in my body do I still feel the imprint of what happened?

What do I wish someone had said to me back then?

Let yourself write the words you needed to hear. Comfort, validation, protection. If no one else said it, say it now — to the version of you who was there.

What do I wish someone had said to me back then?

If I could speak to the person I was just before the birth, what would I say?

This is a sacred kind of time travel. Speak with tenderness. You know now what she didn't. Give her the safety she may not have had.

If I could speak to the person I was just before the birth, what would I say?

TRACING THE TRUTH

SAFETY & FEAR

After trauma, your nervous system can't always distinguish between past danger and present safety. This diagram helps you separate what's safe now from what still feels threatening.

Why it helps:
Seeing your triggers and safe zones side by side helps your nervous system differentiate between threat and safety, empowering you to navigate life with awareness instead of constant hypervigilance.

In the Safe circle, list activities, places, people, or sensations that help you feel grounded.
In the Fear/Trigger circle, list reminders, thoughts, or physical sensations that pull you back into the trauma.

In the overlapping space, write experiences that feel both safe and triggering (e.g., medical appointments that are necessary but anxiety-inducing).

TRACING THE TRUTH

SAFETY & FEAR

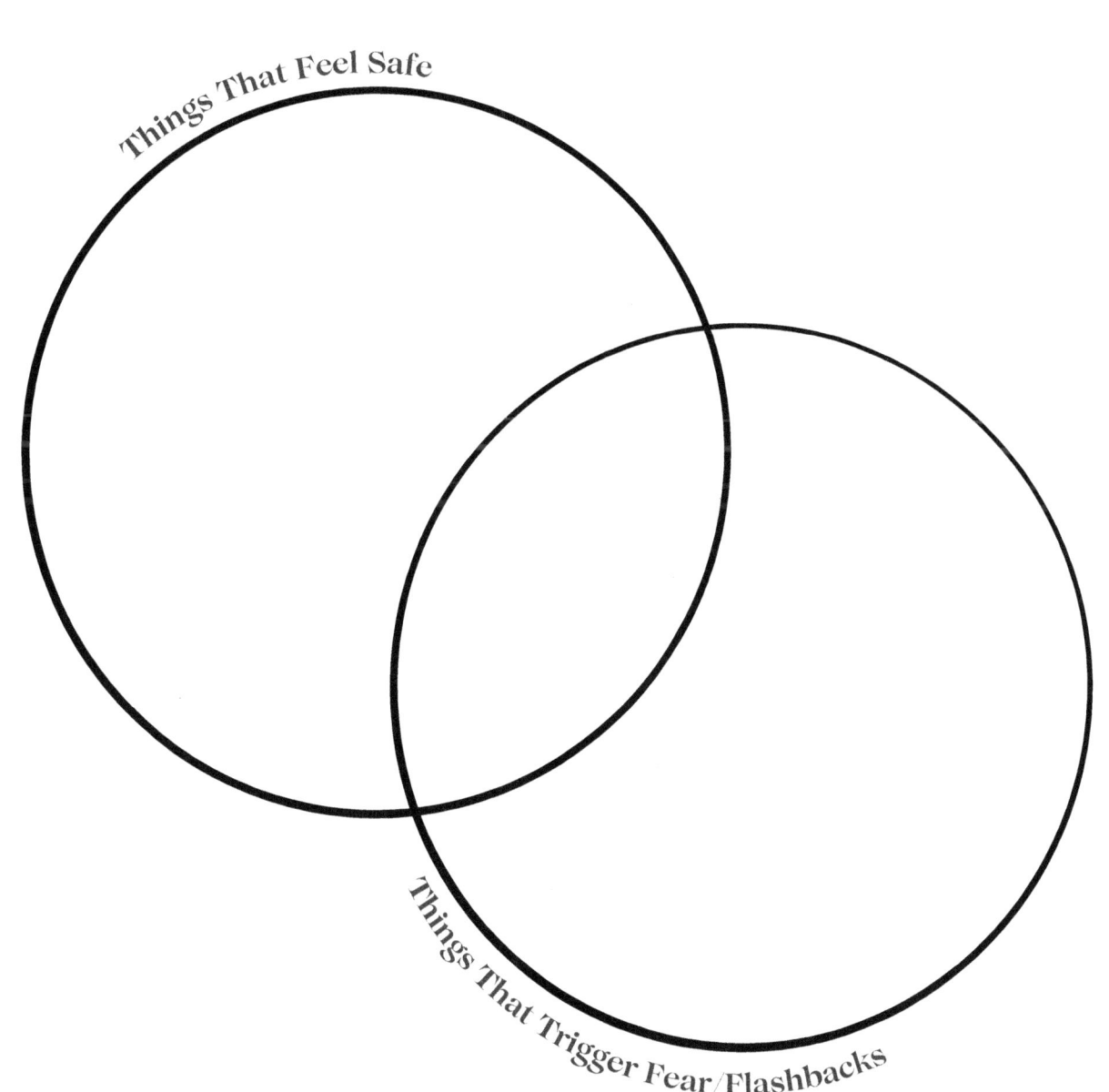

TRACING THE TRUTH

TRAUMA IMPACT TABLE

Birth trauma affects multiple parts of your life—your body, your mind, and your relationships. Seeing it laid out can help you make sense of your experience.

Why it helps:
Visualizing the impact across different domains highlights patterns you might not notice day-to-day. It helps you see that your reactions are normal, connected, and understandable, which is the first step toward reclaiming control and care.

In each column, list ways the trauma shows up.
Be honest and specific: for example, under Body: "heart races at reminders of birth," "stomach tension," "difficulty sleeping."
Under Mind/Emotions: "self-blame," "fear of medical settings."
Under Relationships: "withdrawn from partner," "avoid talking about birth."

Once completed, circle the areas that feel most intense or persistent.

TRACING THE TRUTH

TRAUMA IMPACT TABLE

BODY	MIND/EMOTIONS	RELATIONSHIPS

TRACING THE TRUTH

MAPPING THE IMPRINT

Trauma leaves traces in both mind and body. This exercise helps you notice where your birth experience still lives physically and emotionally, without judgment.

Why it helps:
Mapping the physical imprint of trauma makes the invisible visible. It helps you understand that your reactions are natural, embodied responses, not "failures," and begins a dialogue between your mind and body.

Think about the birth of your child. Then reflect on how you feel and examine the next page.
Mark areas where you feel tension, discomfort, or memories of fear— head, chest, stomach, shoulders, etc.
Next to each area, write the emotions or sensations you notice: "tight," "aching," "numb," "panicked," "cold," etc.

Notice patterns—are certain areas more activated? Are some emotions linked to physical sensations?

TRACING THE TRUTH

MAPPING THE IMPRINT

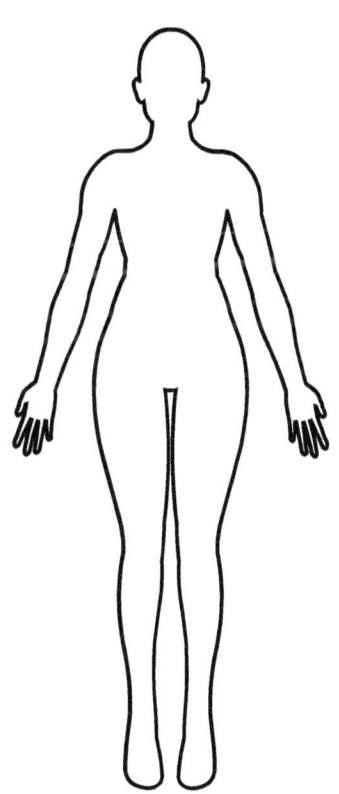

FEELING IN MOTION

Our bodies carry what words often can't — tension, joy, grief, or relief. Moving intentionally helps you process and release emotions stored in the body, while giving a tangible sense of your day's narrative. Ending in a posture of strength signals to your nervous system: I survived, I'm here, I can hold myself steady. This isn't about dancing perfectly or performing for anyone; it's about giving your inner experience a voice through movement, noticing how small gestures can express complex feelings. Over time, this practice reconnects body and mind, helping you feel grounded, seen, and resilient.

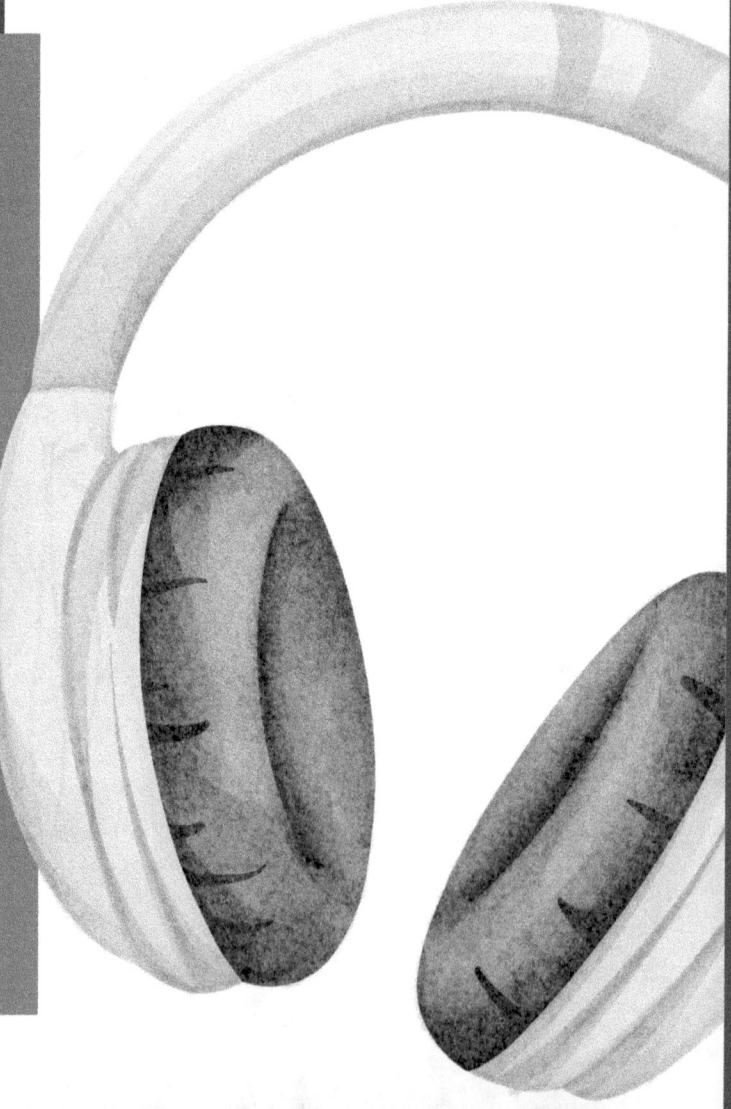

Choose a Song — Something that matches or invites movement for your current state.

Move Freely — Let your body express today's story. Small gestures count — a hand to heart, a sway, a shrug.

Notice — Pay attention to tension, ease, or areas that want attention.

End in Strength — Finish in a posture that conveys groundedness and safety (feet planted, shoulders relaxed, chest open). Hold for 30 seconds.

Reflect — Journal a few words about what your body expressed and how it feels afterward.

ACTION

SAFE STORAGE FOR STRESS

Sometimes our minds replay stress, trauma, or overwhelm on loop. The Container Drawing gives these experiences a safe "home" — a boundary between what's inside and the part of you that is resourced and present. By visualizing a lid you can open only when ready, you create agency over your attention and nervous system. Adding symbols of support reminds your brain that help exists — internal resources, trusted people, or grounding strategies. This isn't avoidance; it's a gentle way to regulate intensity while still acknowledging reality. Over time, your nervous system learns that stress can be noticed without taking over, and you have the tools to manage it.

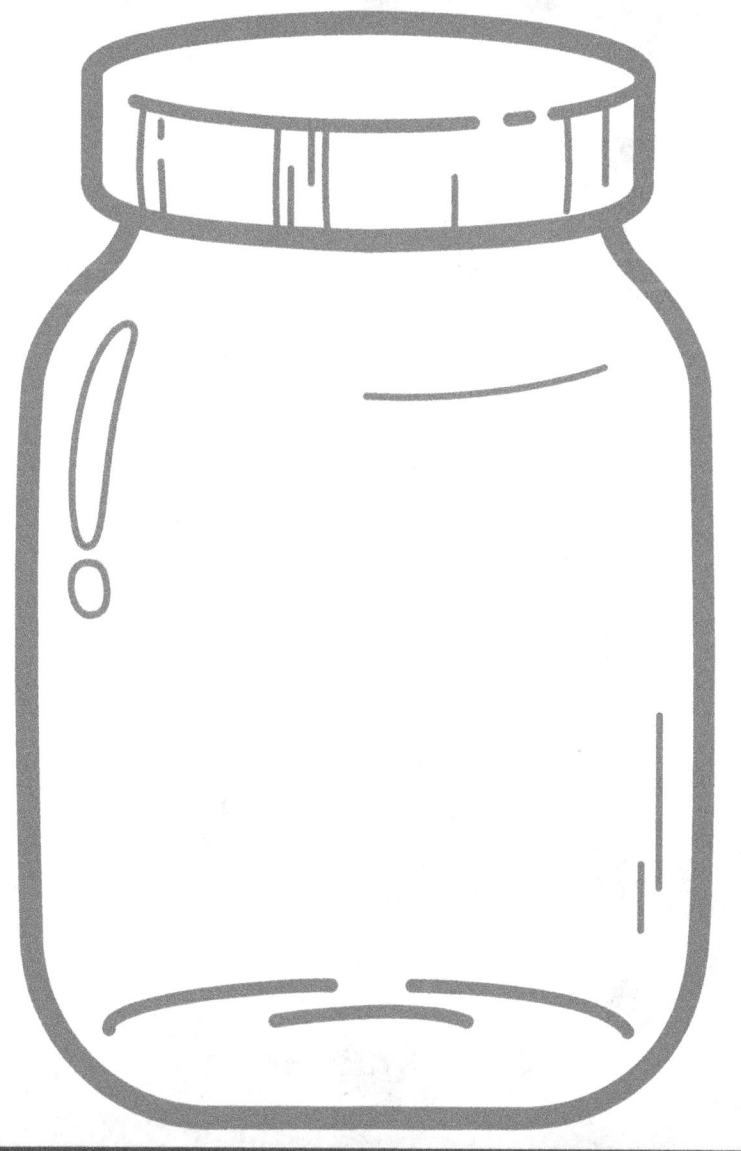

Add Supports — Inside or around the container, draw or list symbols of support (friends, pets, rituals, skills, calming imagery).

Deposit Stress — Place current worries, intrusive thoughts, or tension inside.

Seal the Lid — Draw a lid or closure. Remind yourself: you will open it only when resourced.

Check-In — Practice opening the container gently later, after self-soothing, reflection, or support.

SECTION TWO

The Moment Everything Changed

There's often a moment in trauma — subtle or sharp — when something inside us knows: this isn't okay. It might have been when a decision was made without you. When someone spoke over you. When pain overwhelmed and no one seemed to notice. When time stopped, and your voice disappeared. Trauma doesn't always arrive like a car crash. Sometimes it creeps in through a look, a silence, a sensation your body couldn't process.

This section is here to help you name that moment — or the many moments — without reliving them. Naming is not about rehashing pain. It's about reclaiming power. When we can say, "This is where it hurt," we stop gaslighting ourselves. You're not being dramatic. You're remembering. You're beginning to witness what happened with the support and clarity you might not have had at the time.

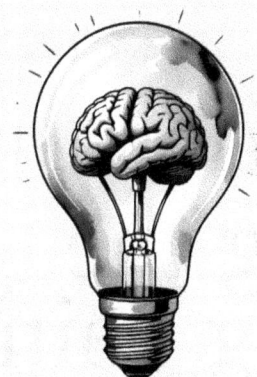

Making Sense Of It
Naming the Turning Point

Trauma doesn't always crash into you like a car accident. Sometimes it creeps in quietly—through a word, a glance, a decision made without you. In birth, that moment can look different for everyone. Maybe it was when the room suddenly felt too bright, too crowded, and you realized no one was listening to you. Maybe it was when pain became unbearable and your pleas for help were ignored. Maybe it was when a doctor or nurse spoke over you, and you felt your voice shrink until it disappeared. There's often a split second, sharp or subtle, when something deep inside whispers: This isn't okay.

That moment matters. It matters because it's the exact point where safety fractured. Birth is supposed to be vulnerable, yes—but not unsafe. And when that boundary is crossed, your whole system responds. Your heart pounds, your body tenses, your sense of control slips away. You might not have named it then—you might have told yourself to push through, to endure—but your body knew. It remembered. That memory doesn't vanish once the baby arrives. It lingers, sometimes buried, sometimes loud, but always present.

Emotionally, this moment leaves a mark because it collides with expectation. We're told birth is supposed to be beautiful, empowering, sacred. So when it turns frightening, lonely, or dehumanizing, the contrast is brutal. You might even gaslight yourself afterward—"Was it really that bad? Should I just be grateful?" But the truth is: naming where it hurt is not being dramatic. It's being honest.

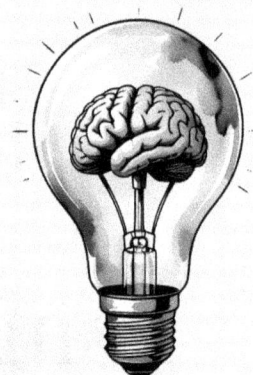

Making Sense Of It
Naming the Turning Point

Socially, it gets even heavier. The world often doesn't make space for women or birthing people to name their trauma. You may hear "At least the baby is healthy" or "All that matters is the outcome." Those phrases, while well-meaning, dismiss the fact that you mattered too. That your safety, your voice, and your experience were just as important as the baby's arrival. When society tells you to "move on," it deepens the wound by denying its reality.

This is why identifying the moment it all changed can feel like both a relief and a rebellion. It breaks the silence. It says: I remember. I was there. And it mattered. You don't have to re-live it in detail. You don't even need the perfect words for it. Simply acknowledging that it existed gives shape to the formless weight you've been carrying. It's like finally saying out loud: This is where it broke. And with that truth, you open the door to healing.

Naming the moment is not about blame. It's about power. It's about reclaiming your right to say what happened to you, in your own language, without shame. It's about giving yourself permission to trust your memory, your body, and your heart again. You deserved safety. You deserved respect. If you didn't get that, the hurt you feel is real.

When did I first feel that something was going wrong?

Was it a look? A word? A change in someone's tone? A medical shift you weren't informed of? Go gently — you're not reliving it, just circling around it from a safe distance.

When did I first feel that something was going wrong?

What do I remember most vividly — and what do I barely remember at all?

Trauma fragments memory. Some things stay too sharp. Others disappear. What's stuck on replay? What's blurry? Let yourself notice without judgment.

What do I remember most vividly — and what do I barely remember at all?

Is there a part of me that still feels frozen in time?

Where in your life — or in your body — do you feel stuck in "the moment"? Can you meet that part with kindness? You're not stuck anymore. But it's okay if it still feels that way.

Is there a part of me that still feels frozen in time?

Who or what made me feel most alone in that experience?

Even in a crowded room, trauma can be lonely. Was there someone who dismissed you? A lack of eye contact? Something that made you feel invisible?

Who or what made me feel most alone in that experience?

What part of me stepped in to survive it?

Did you go numb? Get polite? Push through? Dissociate? This part of you deserves deep respect. You're not weak — you were brilliant at surviving.

What part of me stepped in to survive it?

What do I wish someone had done differently?

Let the truth come out — even if it feels "mean" or "unfair." Anger is often clarity. Write it down as a way of witnessing what you deserved but didn't receive.

What do I wish someone had done differently?

If I could freeze that moment and speak to myself inside it, what would I say?

This is a form of self-rescue. What did that version of you most need to hear or know?

If I could freeze that moment and speak to myself inside it, what would I say?

TRACING THE TRUTH

GIVING LANGUAGE TO SILENCE

Sometimes the wound isn't only what happened, but what didn't — the words left unsaid, the care that never came. Here, you'll give voice to what was missing and begin to offer it back to yourself.

Why it helps:
Trauma often comes from absence — the words or care you didn't receive. By writing and speaking those missing words now, you give your body the affirmation it deserved then. This isn't rewriting history, but offering yourself healing language to close part of the wound.

Take a quiet moment. Imagine yourself in the place where the moment shifted. Without going into every detail, picture yourself there.
Write down the exact words you wish someone had said to you in that moment. Keep it simple, like "You're safe." "We hear you." "We'll slow down." These are words your nervous system longed for.
Now, write down the words that were actually spoken to you — if any. If no one said anything, write "silence."
Compare the two lists. Notice the space between what you needed and what you received.
Place your hand over your heart or belly. Out loud, read the "wish" words slowly, as if speaking them to your past self. You might even close your eyes and imagine whispering them to yourself in that moment.

TRACING THE TRUTH

GIVING LANGUAGE TO SILENCE

What You Wish They Said

What They Actually Said

SELF-COMPASSION BREAK

When stress, shame, or pain flare up, most of us go straight into self-criticism: Why can't I handle this better? What's wrong with me? That inner attack only tightens the spiral. Kristin Neff's Self-Compassion Break interrupts that cycle. It gives you three small handholds: recognition of your pain, the reminder you're not alone in it, and an active choice to soften instead of harden against yourself. With repetition, your nervous system learns that you don't have to white-knuckle through suffering or numb out — you can meet yourself with the same tenderness you'd extend to a friend. That shift doesn't erase the pain, but it changes the way it lands in your body. Over time, it builds resilience, because you're no longer abandoned in hard moments; you become your own safe ally.

Notice —
Pause and acknowledge: "This is hard. This hurts."

Kindness —
Place a hand on your chest or cheek and whisper: "May I be gentle with myself right now."

Common Humanity —
Say: "Others feel this too. I'm not the only one struggling."

POCKET MOOD LIFTERS

When life feels heavy, it's easy to forget what actually helps. In hard moments, the brain tends to focus on what's wrong, not what's available. An Antidote List is your preloaded reminder: ten small, proven things that shift your state even a little. These aren't grand fixes or instant cures — they're micro-adjustments that keep you from sliding deeper into the stuckness. Pairing an antidote before a hard task helps you face it with steadier energy; using one after provides recovery and closure so you don't carry the weight forward. Over time, this list becomes muscle memory — your nervous system learns, When I struggle, I have options. That's the opposite of hopelessness.

1 **List Ten** — Write down 10 things that reliably lift your mood (a song, a walk, fresh air, texting a safe friend, lighting a candle). Keep them small and doable.

....

....

....

....

....

....

....

2 **Use Before** — Pick one before facing a task you tend to dread. Let it soften resistance.

3 **Use After** — Choose another as a closing ritual. Let it tell your body, That part is done. I'm safe again.

ACTION

ENERGY BUDGET

Energy is a limited resource, and most of us spend it like it's endless. By mapping your natural peaks and dips, you begin treating energy the same way you'd treat money — something to spend with intention. Research shows that syncing meaningful tasks with your personal rhythms increases follow-through and reduces burnout. Protecting a rest block is equally vital. Too often, rest is treated as optional, the first thing cut when life gets busy. But rest is where your nervous system resets and your resilience stores refill. By scheduling it like a non-negotiable meeting, you reclaim the truth that your wellbeing is not secondary — it's the foundation.

Map Peaks + Valleys — Track when you feel most alert and when you feel sluggish over 2–3 days. Note the times.

Match Tasks — Place your most meaningful or demanding actions inside your natural energy peaks. Save automatic or lighter tasks for your dips.

Schedule Rest — Block at least one daily rest period (nap, walk, quiet time). Treat it as sacred — no canceling, no apologizing.

ENERGY BUDGET

Energy is a limited resource, and most of us spend it like it's endless. By mapping your natural peaks and dips, you begin treating energy the same way you'd treat money — something to spend with intention. Research shows that syncing meaningful tasks with your personal rhythms increases follow-through and reduces burnout. Protecting a rest block is equally vital. Too often, rest is treated as optional, the first thing cut when life gets busy. But rest is where your nervous system resets and your resilience stores refill. By scheduling it like a non-negotiable meeting, you reclaim the truth that your wellbeing is not secondary — it's the foundation.

Map Peaks + Valleys — Track when you feel most alert and when you feel sluggish over 2–3 days. Note the times.

Match Tasks — Place your most meaningful or demanding actions inside your natural energy peaks. Save automatic or lighter tasks for your dips.

Schedule Rest — Block at least one daily rest period (nap, walk, quiet time). Treat it as sacred — no canceling, no apologizing.

Time	Feeling	Tasks	Notes

ENERGY BUDGET

Time	Feeling	Tasks	Notes

SECTION THREE

When My Body Wasn't Safe Anymore

For many people who go through birth trauma, the body becomes a confusing, even frightening place afterward. The same body that carried life may now feel foreign. You might flinch from touch, experience flashbacks, carry tension or pain, or feel completely numb. And it's not just about physical recovery — it's about safety. Safety in your own skin. Safety when you close your eyes. Safety when someone says, "You're okay now," and your body whispers back, "No, I'm not."

This section isn't here to fix your body — because your body was never broken. It's here to help you listen to it again. To gently rebuild trust with the place where your trauma was stored. The body is where we carry everything that wasn't allowed to be felt or expressed. You don't need to force anything — we're just beginning to ask, "What are you holding?" and "Can I be with you, kindly?" This is the first step to coming home to yourself.

Making Sense Of It
When the Body Stops Feeling Like Home

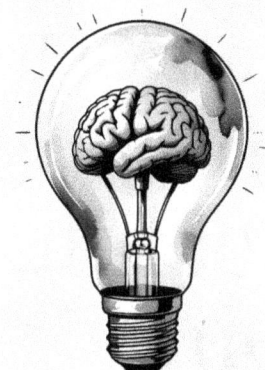

When birth trauma happens, it doesn't just leave a memory — it lives in the body. The place that carried life, endured hours of effort, and was supposed to feel like your sanctuary can suddenly feel unrecognizable. Many people describe this shift as if their body has turned against them. The same arms that once cradled, the same heart that beat through contractions, the same skin that stretched to hold another life — now feels foreign, unsafe, or unbearable to inhabit.

It's important to understand why this happens. Trauma isn't stored as a neat story in the mind. It lodges itself in sensations, reflexes, and responses. The nervous system, whose entire job is to keep you alive, takes note of everything: the moment you felt ignored, the second pain became too much, the instant a voice told you, you're fine when you knew you weren't. In that split second, your body concluded: I'm not safe here. From that point forward, your body responded accordingly — tightening, bracing, numbing, or flinching at even the hint of danger.

Think of your body as a house. Before trauma, it was imperfect but familiar. Maybe there were creaky floors or doors that stuck, but it was home. Then, during birth, the walls cracked. Maybe someone stormed in without asking. Maybe the lights flickered and went out. Maybe the foundation shook so hard you thought the whole structure would collapse. After that, of course you'd hesitate to walk back inside. Of course you'd question if this house — your body — could protect you again.

Making Sense Of It
When the Body Stops Feeling Like Home

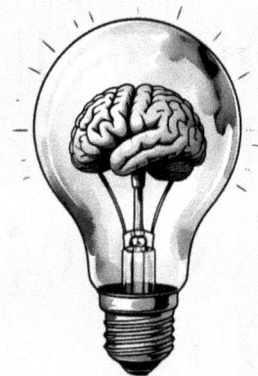

And yet, that house still stands. Even in its shaken state, it has been protecting you in the only way it knows how. Every panic response, every ache that won't ease, every moment of disconnection — it's not your body failing you. It's your body saying: I am guarding the place where it all happened. Survival is not betrayal. Your body did what it needed to do to get you through.

But here's the other truth: just as your body holds onto trauma, it also holds onto safety, love, and resilience. Think about the times you laughed so hard your belly hurt, the warmth of a hug that melted your shoulders, or the rhythm of your breath when you finally felt at ease. Those moments are stored in your body too. Trauma might feel louder right now, but it doesn't erase what was good.

Healing begins not by silencing your body, but by listening to it differently. By saying: I see you. I know why you're bracing. I know why you're holding. It means treating your body less like an enemy and more like a child who's been through something unbearable — a child who needs safety, patience, and tenderness before they'll trust again.

What has changed in how I feel in my body since the birth?

Be honest. Is there fear? Anger? Detachment? A new kind of pain or tightness? A way you avoid looking in the mirror or being touched? Your honesty here is already healing.

What has changed in how I feel in my body since the birth?

What does "safety" feel like — and where do I notice its absence?

When was the last time you felt safe in your body — even for a moment? Where do you feel unsafe now? Notice without judgment. Naming it brings it out of hiding.

What does "safety" feel like — and where do I notice its absence?

What is my body trying to tell me that I haven't wanted to hear?

Sometimes the body speaks in symptoms, sensations, or silence. If you asked your body directly, "What are you holding for me?" — what might it say?

What is my body trying to tell me that I haven't wanted to hear?

Are there parts of my body I avoid or feel shame around now?

This is so common and so tender. If there's a part of your body that feels "ruined" or painful to acknowledge, you are not alone. Let yourself name it gently.

Are there parts of my body I avoid or feel shame around now?

If my body could speak without being interrupted, what would it say?

Try free-writing as if your body had a voice — without your mind filtering it. What does it need? What is it still afraid of? What is it proud of?

If my body could speak without being interrupted, what would it say?

What would rebuilding trust with my body look like — one small step at a time?

Could it be one breath? One hand over your heart? One moment of stillness? You don't have to rush. Trust is built slowly, and you get to decide how.

What would rebuilding trust with my body look like — one small step at a time?

ACTION

ORIENTATION

When anxiety or overwhelm spikes, the mind and body can feel unmoored, as if you're "floating" in your thoughts. Orientation gently reconnects you with your environment, reminding your nervous system that you are safe in this moment. Slowly scanning your surroundings with your eyes and naming what you notice allows your body to register the present physically, which can reduce hypervigilance, grounding you in both sight and sensation.

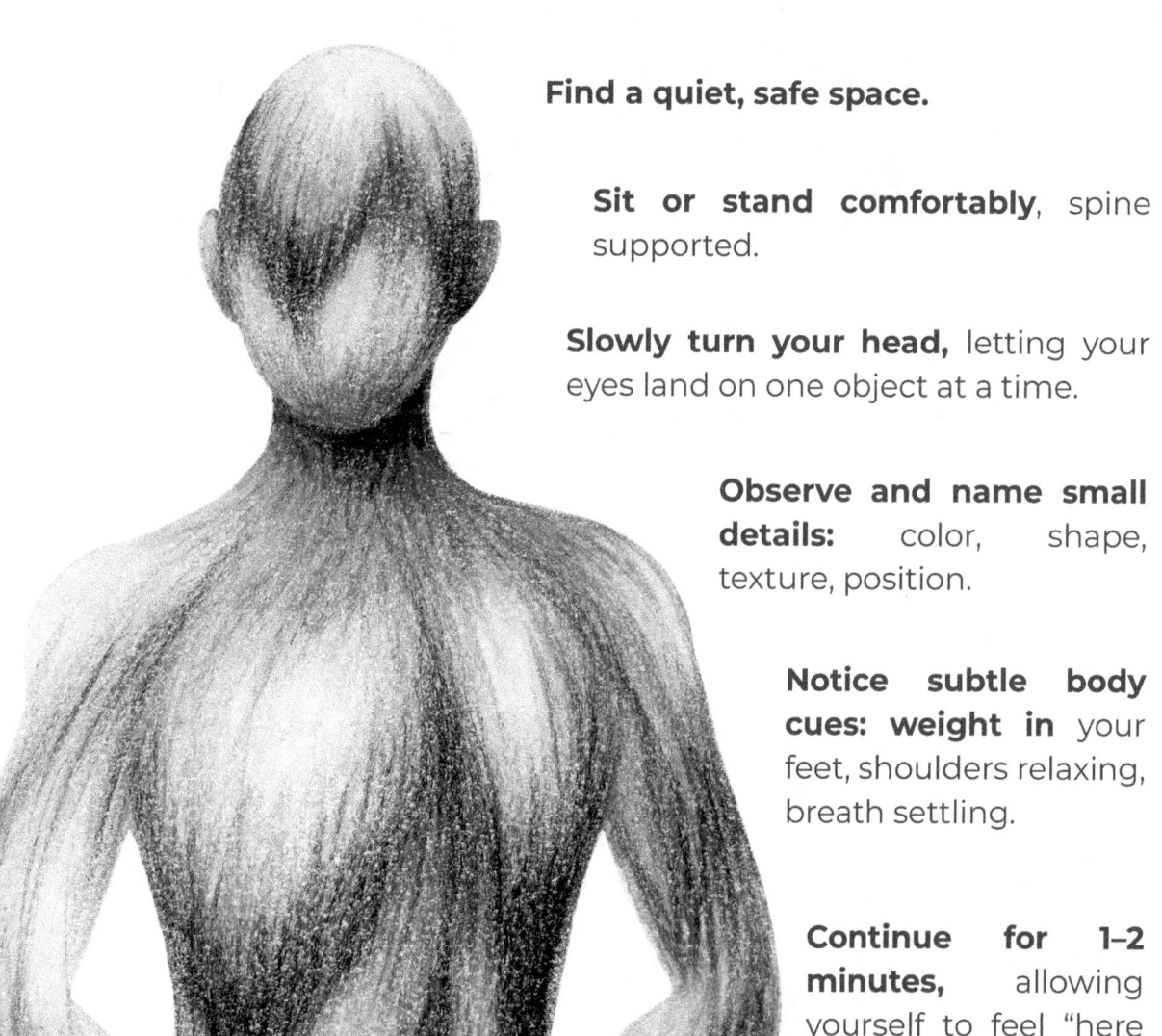

Find a quiet, safe space.

Sit or stand comfortably, spine supported.

Slowly turn your head, letting your eyes land on one object at a time.

Observe and name small details: color, shape, texture, position.

Notice subtle body cues: weight in your feet, shoulders relaxing, breath settling.

Continue for 1–2 minutes, allowing yourself to feel "here and now."

SECTION FOUR

The Aftershock – When Everyone Moved On but I Couldn't

There comes a strange moment after trauma when the room clears. The appointments stop. The phone calls slow down. People expect you to smile again, to be "grateful it's over." But what they don't see is that you're still in it. Inside, the aftershocks are still shaking you. You may look "recovered," but your nervous system hasn't landed. Your heart hasn't caught up. Your spirit is still stuck in the hallway between crisis and healing, waiting for someone to say, "It makes sense you're still not okay."

This chapter is a space for what happens after. For the slow unraveling. For the grief that didn't fit the calendar. You're not broken for taking longer. You're not dramatic for still feeling what others have dismissed. You're simply a human whose pain wasn't witnessed long enough. And in these pages, we stay with that pain — not to wallow in it, but to honor what your system needed... and still needs.

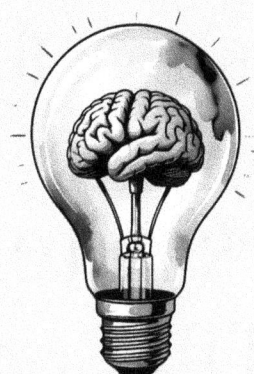

Making Sense Of It
Living in the Tremors After the Storm

The world loves a clean ending. Baby's born, you're home, the crisis is "over." People want the tidy story: the mother survives, the child survives, the family moves on. But trauma doesn't obey that narrative. For so many, the hardest part isn't the birth itself — it's the silence that follows. The moment the noise dies down and you're left alone with the aftershocks pulsing through your body.

Think of an earthquake. Buildings can look intact from the outside, but step inside and you see the cracks: beams shifted, foundations unstable, things rattling loose long after the shaking stops. That's what birth trauma feels like. The world might look at you and think, She's fine now. But your nervous system is still quivering. Your emotions are still braced for impact. You are still living inside the aftershock.

Here's the raw truth: our culture doesn't give women or birthing people enough space for aftermath. There are appointments for stitches and blood pressure, but not for the invisible fracture of trust in your body. There's a check-up for the baby's weight, but not for the weight sitting in your chest. The expectation is that you've "moved on," when in reality, you're only beginning to process what happened.

The aftershock is confusing because it doesn't always announce itself with screams or tears. Sometimes it's quiet. Numbness. Dissociation.

Making Sense Of It
Living in the Tremors After the Storm

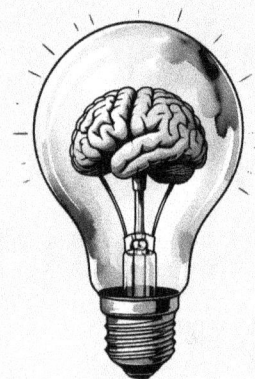

A sudden flood of panic when you hear a hospital monitor beep. The way your body tenses before sleep, as though it's still waiting for something to go wrong. These aren't signs that you're broken — they're signs that your nervous system is still protecting you. It hasn't yet received the message: The danger has passed. This is why the aftershock can feel lonelier than the trauma itself. During the crisis, at least people could see you were suffering. But in the aftermath, you're expected to wear normalcy like a costume while your insides keep trembling. That gap — between how the world sees you and how you actually feel — can be its own kind of wound.

But here's the invitation: what if the aftershock isn't failure? What if it's evidence of your survival? Every tremor is your body saying, I am still here. I am still processing. I'm still trying to protect you. Instead of fighting those ripples, what if you met them with curiosity? What if you honored them as the language of healing, not the proof of damage?

You don't need to rush past this part. The aftershock is not weakness; it's simply your system recalibrating. Healing isn't about snapping your fingers and being "fine." It's about giving yourself permission to feel the reverberations — and to trust that eventually, with time and compassion, the ground will steady again.

You are not behind. You are not failing. You are simply living in the space between survival and peace. And that space is valid. It is human. And it deserves to be honored.

What did people stop asking about — even though I was still hurting?

Reflect on what felt dropped too soon. Were you still in pain while others moved on? What conversations were silenced before you were ready?

What did people stop asking about — even though I was still hurting?

What parts of me felt abandoned once the immediate crisis ended?

Was it your emotional self? Your spiritual sense of meaning? Your body? Describe the places in you that felt left behind.

What parts of me felt abandoned once the immediate crisis ended?

What do I wish someone had said — even just once?

Sometimes healing begins with imagining the words we never heard. Let yourself write out the sentences that would have brought relief or validation.

What do I wish someone had said — even just once?

What's the cost of pretending I'm "okay" when I'm not?

Many people wear masks after trauma just to function. What has that cost you — emotionally, physically, relationally?

What's the cost of pretending I'm "okay" when I'm not?

What still needs to be witnessed, even now?

Is there a part of your story, body, or spirit that no one really looked at? That deserves presence, even today? Give that space on the page.

What still needs to be witnessed, even now?

How would I show up differently if I didn't have to rush my healing?

Explore what your grief or trauma would look like with permission. Slower? Gentler? More supported?

How would I show up differently if I didn't have to rush my healing?

TRACING THE TRUTH

TIMELINE OF THE LINGERING

Trauma doesn't always end when the event is over. This exercise helps you honor the moments your nervous system is still processing.

Why it helps:
Seeing the timeline helps you validate that your healing isn't linear, and that lingering reactions aren't a sign of weakness—they're proof your system is still catching up.

On a blank page, draw a horizontal line representing "the day of birth trauma" on the left and "today" on the right.
Along the line, mark moments, feelings, or sensations that still hit you unexpectedly — flashbacks, sudden panic, physical tension, or intrusive thoughts.
Write a brief note about what each moment felt like and how your body responded.

TRACING THE TRUTH

TIMELINE OF THE LINGERING

TRACING THE TRUTH

LETTER TO THE WORLD THAT MOVED ON

Sometimes the people around us — friends, family, doctors, society — move on while we are still inside the storm. This exercise is about giving voice to what wasn't seen, held, or acknowledged.

Why it helps:
Naming the unseen grief gives it form. Even if others cannot hold it, you can witness your own experience and reclaim your story.

Choose someone, or even a collective "you" — a doctor, nurse, partner, friend, or society at large.
Use these prompts if you want:
"You thought I was okay, but what you didn't see was…"
"I needed you to stay longer because…"
"It wasn't over for me, and here's why…"
"I still carry ___, and it deserves to be witnessed."
Write without censoring. No need to be polite. No need to protect anyone else's feelings.
Close with a line of truth: "Even if they couldn't stay, I am staying with myself now."
Decide what to do with your letter: burn it (safely), bury it, keep it somewhere sacred, or share it with someone safe.

TRACING THE TRUTH

LETTER TO THE WORLD THAT MOVED ON

TRACING THE TRUTH

LETTER TO THE WORLD THAT MOVED ON

TRACING THE TRUTH

LETTER TO THE WORLD THAT MOVED ON

TRACING THE TRUTH

LETTER TO THE WORLD THAT MOVED ON

WORRY WINDOW

Worries often hijack your mind, showing up at every unexpected moment. By giving them a dedicated "time slot," you reclaim control instead of letting them run your day. This practice teaches your nervous system that there's a safe space and a safe time to process, so you're not constantly reacting to every intrusive thought. During the window, you can gently evaluate what's actionable versus what you need to let go, building clarity and self-trust. Outside the window, a simple cue like "not now—later" helps you return to the present without guilt or shame. Over time, this simple structure reduces the intensity and frequency of anxious loops.

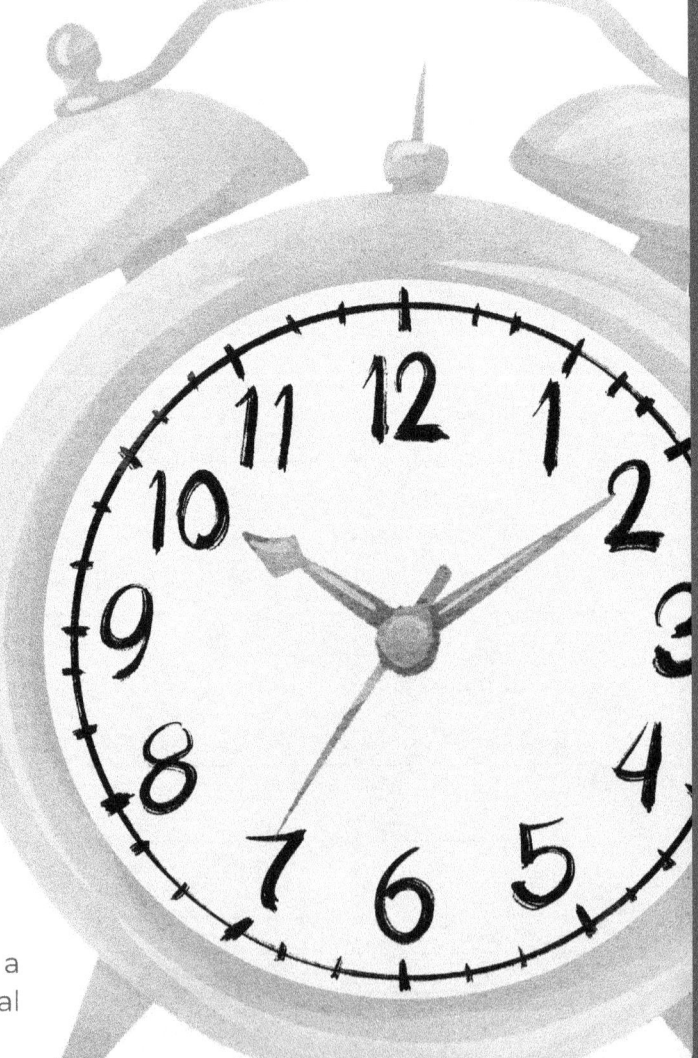

Park your worries: Write them down as they arise.

....

....

....

....

Set a 15-minute window: Choose a consistent time each day for processing.

....

Outside the window: Use a cue phrase like "not now—later" to return to your day.

Inside the window: Review the list. Solve what's actionable, accept what isn't, and release judgment.

Close the window: End with a grounding or soothing activity to signal completion.

GENTLE BREATH FOCUS

When anxiety spikes, the mind and body race together — thoughts accelerate, heart rate climbs, muscles tighten. Counting your breath gives both something steady to follow. By pairing inhale and exhale with numbers, you create a gentle anchor that slows the nervous system, refocuses attention, and interrupts spiraling thoughts. This isn't about perfection or achieving ten — it's about returning to the rhythm whenever distraction occurs. Even a few minutes daily strengthens your capacity to notice tension, settle your body, and move through anxious moments with less overwhelm.

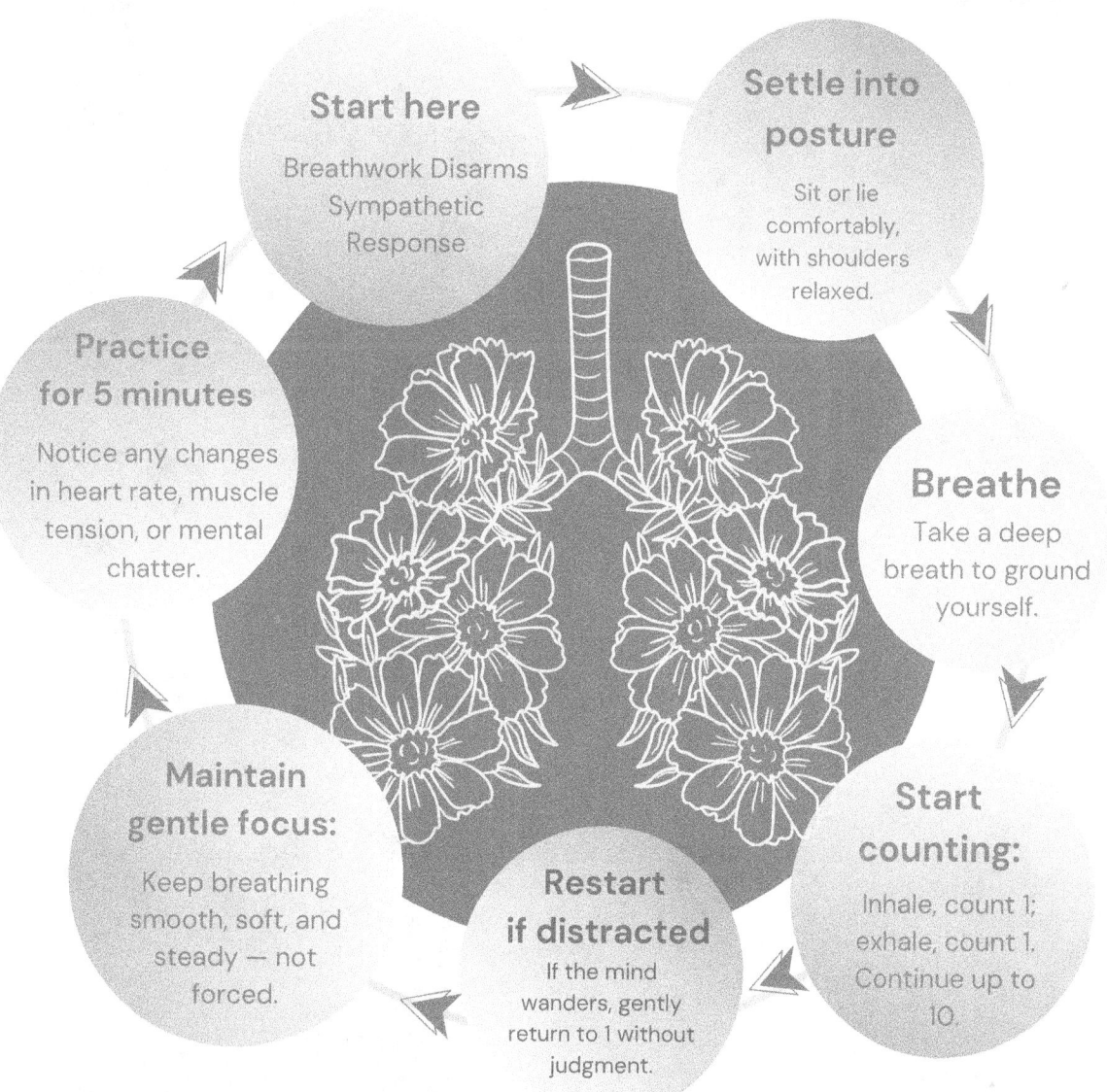

SECTION FIVE

Touch, Sex, and Sensitivity – When Intimacy Feels Impossible

Trauma doesn't stay neatly in the past. It lingers in muscles that flinch at touch, in skin that once welcomed affection but now pulls away. After birth trauma, the body often becomes a stranger — or worse, a battleground. Many people feel ashamed that sex doesn't feel the same, or that touch triggers anxiety instead of closeness. You might wonder if you're broken. You're not. You're surviving.

This chapter is a permission slip to name what often goes unspoken: that intimacy can feel threatening, overwhelming, or simply unwanted. This isn't about fixing you — it's about understanding what your nervous system is trying to say. Your sensitivity is not a failure of love. It's a call for gentleness, patience, and rebuilding safety from the inside out. This space is here to help you reconnect — not just with a partner, but with yourself. Slowly. Tenderly. On your terms.

Making Sense Of It
When Intimacy Feels Impossible

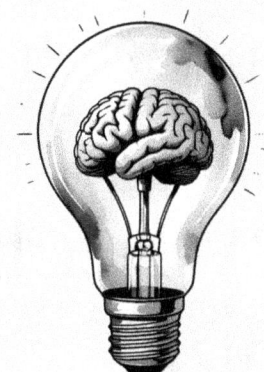

Intimacy after birth trauma is rarely as simple as "getting back to normal." It's not just a matter of desire or attraction; it's about the complex, invisible dialogue between your nervous system, your memories, your body, and the culture you live in. Trauma lives in tissues, in breath, in the tiny reflexes and sensations that your conscious mind can't always control. The very body that brought life into the world — or was present during the attempt to do so — may now feel foreign, unpredictable, or even unsafe. Your skin, once a conduit of pleasure or comfort, may feel like a map of what happened, etched with tension, fear, and survival instincts.

Psychologically, this is about more than just fear. Trauma rewires the nervous system in a way that prioritizes protection over pleasure. The fight-flight-freeze responses that helped you survive a terrifying or disempowering birth don't automatically switch off afterward. A touch that once signaled safety can now trigger hypervigilance; a gentle hug can feel like an invasion. Shame compounds this. Society often tells you that "sex should feel good," that "intimacy fixes everything," or that "you should just be grateful your baby is here." These messages ignore the reality that your body is carrying memory in ways that no amount of rational reassurance can instantly undo. Feeling disconnected, anxious, or numb in intimate moments is not evidence of brokenness — it is evidence of a body and mind doing their job: keeping you safe.

Sociologically, birth and postpartum experiences are wrapped in expectations.

Making Sense Of It
When Intimacy Feels Impossible

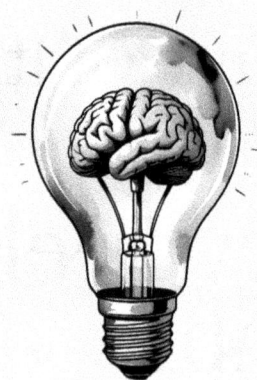

We're taught that mothers should recover quickly, that closeness and sex should resume according to some invisible timeline, and that expressing fear or hesitation is a weakness. These societal pressures can isolate you, making you feel abnormal, ashamed, or defective. Anthropologically, many cultures recognize the postpartum period as sacred — a time for rest, recuperation, and gradual reintegration into social and sexual life. In our modern context, we've lost much of that communal support, and instead, we are expected to perform "normalcy" while negotiating deep psychological and bodily ruptures alone.

The key to rebuilding intimacy is understanding that sex and touch are not the problem — trauma is. Sensitivity, avoidance, or ambivalence around touch are survival responses, not failures. Healing begins by redefining what safety, closeness, and desire mean for you. This requires listening to your body without judgment, honoring its boundaries, and cultivating experiences of consent, pleasure, and connection on your own timeline. It's about negotiating with your nervous system, one breath and one boundary at a time, until touch can exist as a choice rather than a trigger.

Intimacy in this context becomes less about performance and more about attunement: noticing what feels safe, asking for what you need, and allowing desire to re-emerge organically.

Making Sense Of It
When Intimacy Feels Impossible

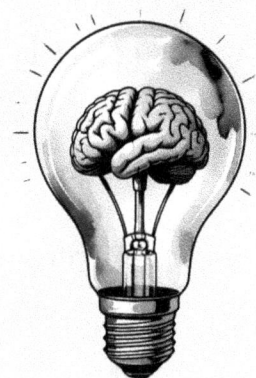

Reconnecting sexually or sensually does not mean erasing the trauma — it means coexisting with it while reclaiming your body as yours again. It's a slow, layered process, informed by the way our bodies encode memory, the social expectations imposed on mothers, and the very real ways culture shapes our sense of shame, autonomy, and worth. In reclaiming touch and intimacy, you're not just surviving; you are asserting agency, rewriting what closeness can be, and honoring your body as a living record of both trauma and resilience.

Your nervous system has learned lessons about danger, loss, and betrayal — now it needs lessons in trust, safety, and consent. That education doesn't happen overnight, but every small moment of connection, every boundary you honor, every experience of pleasure or comfort is a reclamation of yourself. This is what it means to be human after trauma: negotiating between fear and desire, history and possibility, protection and pleasure. And in that negotiation, you are learning not just to survive, but to inhabit your body fully, tenderly, and on your own terms.

How has my relationship with touch changed since the trauma?

Explore what kinds of touch feel safe, unsafe, confusing, or absent now. Be specific. No judgment.

How has my relationship with touch changed since the trauma?

What does my body need before it can feel safe with someone else?

Think about pace, space, voice tone, lighting, physical environment. What helps you feel more in control?

What does my body need before it can feel safe with someone else?

What messages have I received about what sex "should" be like — and how do those messages make me feel now?

Gently challenge internalized expectations. Name where shame might be rooted.

What messages have I received about what sex "should" be like — and how do those messages make me feel now?

In what ways have I felt pressure to "get back to normal"?

Name where you've felt rushed — by a partner, culture, or even yourself.

In what ways have I felt pressure to "get back to normal"?

Can I remember a time my body felt like mine — or imagine what that might feel like again?

Use imagery or memory. What would reclaiming your body look like on your own terms?

Can I remember a time my body felt like mine — or imagine what that might feel like again?

Where do I need permission to say "no" — or "not yet"?

Reflect on where consent has been murky or overridden, and what boundaries your body might be asking for now.

Where do I need permission to say "no" — or "not yet"?

TRACING THE TRUTH

THE COMFORT & TRIGGER MAP

After birth trauma, your body may hold memories in subtle or obvious ways. This exercise helps you visualize where your body feels safe, neutral, or triggered, and begins to untangle the emotional weight tied to touch. It's a non-verbal way of communicating with yourself — giving clarity to your body's signals so you can reconnect on your own terms.

Why it helps:
This visual exercise externalizes internal experiences, giving language to what often feels invisible. It allows you to track progress over time, notice small shifts toward safety, and communicate needs with partners or therapists without relying solely on words.

Use the next page for the outline of your body.
Use colors or symbols to mark areas that feel:
Safe / Comfortable
Neutral / Mixed
Triggered / Uncomfortable
Reflect: Are there patterns? Are certain areas associated with memories, fear, or past trauma?
Journal briefly about what surprised you, what you expected, and what you feel ready to explore.

TRACING THE TRUTH

THE COMFORT & TRIGGER MAP

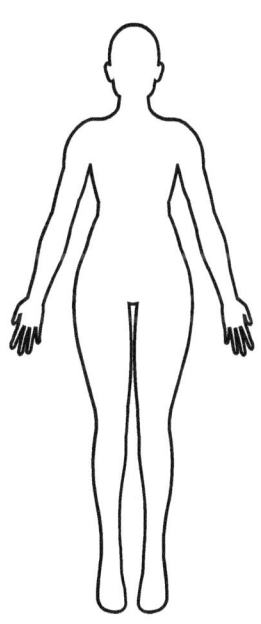

TRACING THE TRUTH

THE COMFORT & TRIGGER MAP

TRACING THE TRUTH

YOUR INTIMACY LETTER

After birth trauma, intimacy can feel complicated, confusing, or even frightening. Writing a letter allows you to give voice to what's often unspoken — your fears, your boundaries, your needs — without needing to perform or justify yourself in the moment. This exercise isn't about educating anyone unless you want to; it's about honoring your experience and creating clarity for yourself first.

Why it helps:
Writing externalizes complex emotions, creating clarity in a space that may otherwise feel confusing. It validates your lived experience, reduces internal conflict, and strengthens communication — first with yourself, then with others. By putting words to what often feels invisible, you reclaim authority over your body, your boundaries, and your emotional landscape.

Address the letter — it can be to a partner, future partner, or even to yourself. Begin with your truth:
"This is what I need you to know about why I've changed..."
"Touch feels different for me now because..."
"I may need more time, patience, or space, and that's not a reflection of my love..."
Name emotions without apology: Share fear, anxiety, shame, or avoidance openly. Include moments when intimacy felt unsafe, overwhelming, or triggering.
Express your boundaries and needs: *"I need...", "I feel safest when...", "It helps me when you..."* This creates concrete steps for communication without judgment.
Close with self-compassion: Acknowledge your resilience: "I am allowed to feel this way. I am rebuilding trust with my body and my heart at my own pace."

TRACING THE TRUTH

YOUR INTIMACY LETTER

TRACING THE TRUTH

YOUR INTIMACY LETTER

ACTION

PROGRESSIVE MUSCLE RELAXATION

When stress lingers, tension builds in muscles without us noticing, keeping the nervous system on high alert. PMR gently signals to your body that it's safe to let go. By intentionally tensing and then releasing each muscle group, you highlight the difference between tension and relaxation, training your body to notice and release stress. This practice doesn't just relax the muscles—it communicates to your nervous system that it can downshift, making calm feel real and accessible.

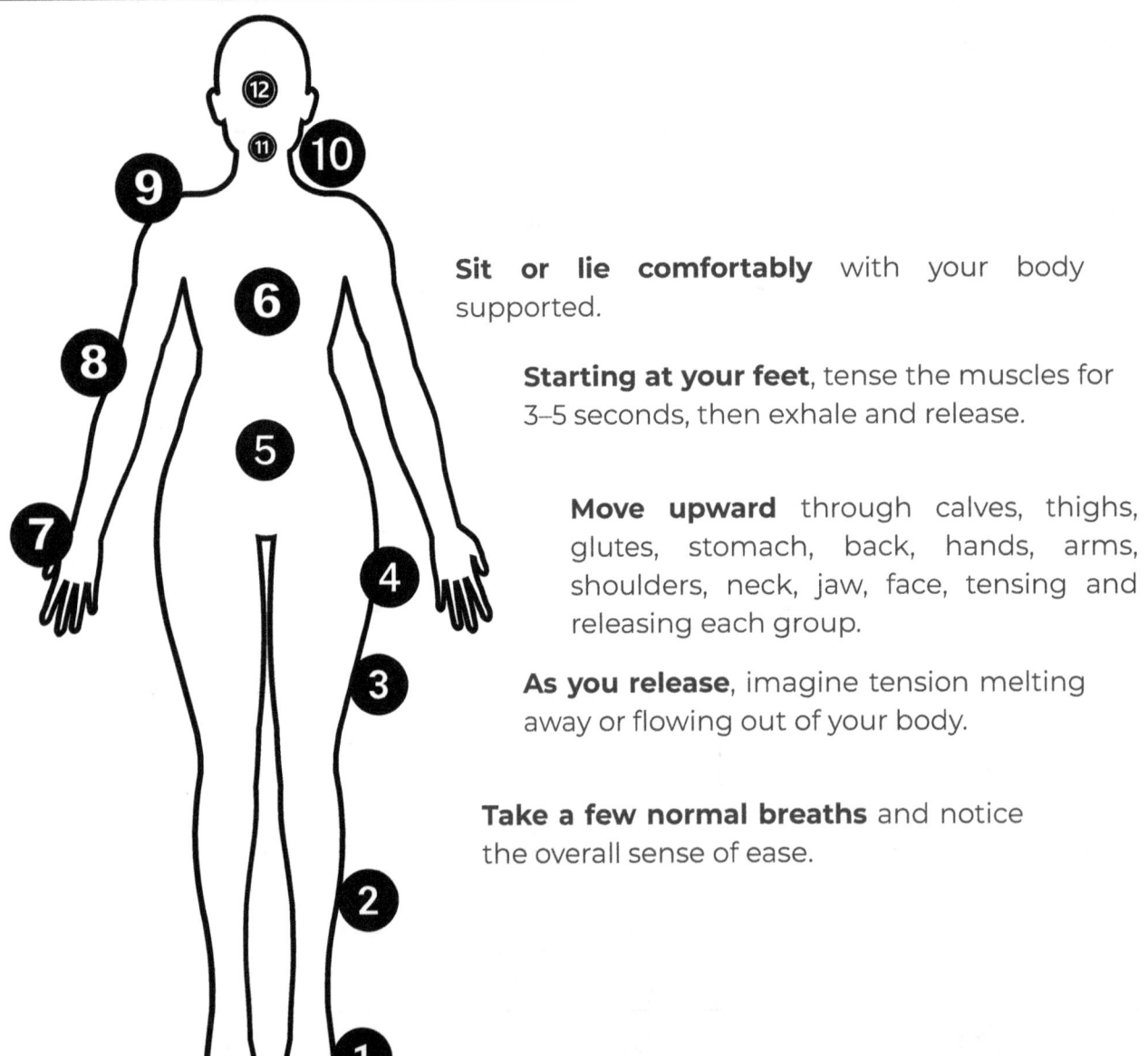

Sit or lie comfortably with your body supported.

Starting at your feet, tense the muscles for 3–5 seconds, then exhale and release.

Move upward through calves, thighs, glutes, stomach, back, hands, arms, shoulders, neck, jaw, face, tensing and releasing each group.

As you release, imagine tension melting away or flowing out of your body.

Take a few normal breaths and notice the overall sense of ease.

ACTION

THE VOO RESET

Our vagus nerve connects the brain and body, regulating stress and calm. Gentle vocalization, like a long "voo" on the exhale, stimulates this pathway, sending a signal that it's safe to downshift arousal. The vibration through your chest and throat also grounds your attention in your body, giving your nervous system tangible proof that it can relax. Just a few rounds can reduce tension, slow your heart rate, and invite a sense of ease.

Sit or stand comfortably with shoulders relaxed.

Inhale slowly through your nose.

Exhale while vocalizing a long, gentle "voo," letting your chest and throat vibrate.

Repeat for 3 rounds, noticing the sensations and any shift in tension.

Place a hand on your chest to feel the vibration more clearly.

SECTION SIX

What Happened to Me? Making Sense of the Medical Mayhem

Sometimes the hardest part of birth trauma is that it all happened so fast — or so confusingly — that you can't even put the pieces together. You might have been told everything was "fine." Maybe your chart says "routine." But inside, you know something wasn't right. Whether it was the rushed decisions, ignored instincts, cold hands, or the way no one looked you in the eye — your body remembers.

This chapter is here to help you gently untangle the knot of what happened, what it meant, and how it left its mark. Not for the sake of reliving it — but to validate what your body already knows, and to begin rebuilding a sense of agency. When systems fail to explain or acknowledge trauma, our healing begins when we dare to name it ourselves. This is your space to reclaim the story — not the one they wrote down, but the one your soul lived.

Making Sense Of It
Healing After Medical Birth Trauma

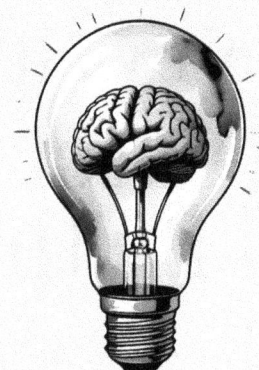

Birth trauma often unfolds in a setting that is supposed to be a sanctuary — a place where life is brought into the world with care and expertise. Yet, for many, the hospital becomes a place of fear, confusion, and betrayal. The sterile environment, the cold machinery, the rushed decisions — all of these can transform what should be a sacred experience into a traumatic ordeal.

In the aftermath, it's common to feel a profound sense of loss — not just of control, but of trust. Trust in the medical system, in healthcare providers, and perhaps most painfully, in your own body. When you were told everything was "fine," yet your body remembers otherwise, it creates a chasm between your lived experience and the narrative imposed upon you.

This disconnect can lead to a cascade of emotions: anger at being dismissed, fear of future medical encounters, and a deep sense of vulnerability. The very tools designed to aid you — monitors, IVs, surgical instruments — may now evoke anxiety or panic. The sounds of beeping machines can trigger a rush of memories, and the sight of a white coat can send your heart racing.

But it's important to understand that these reactions are valid. They are the echoes of a system that failed to honor your humanity, your autonomy, and your voice. Your trauma is not a result of over-sensitivity; it is a legitimate response to being treated as a case rather than a person.

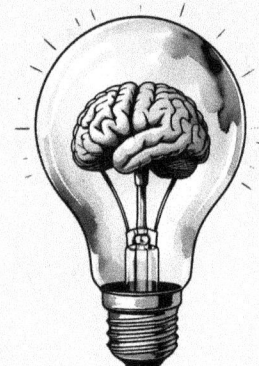

Making Sense Of It
Healing After Medical Birth Trauma

Birth trauma often unfolds in a setting that is supposed to be a sanctuary — a place where life is brought into the world with care and expertise. Yet, for many, the hospital becomes a place of fear, confusion, and betrayal. The sterile environment, the cold machinery, the rushed decisions — all of these can transform what should be a sacred experience into a traumatic ordeal.

In the aftermath, it's common to feel a profound sense of loss — not just of control, but of trust. Trust in the medical system, in healthcare providers, and perhaps most painfully, in your own body. When you were told everything was "fine," yet your body remembers otherwise, it creates a chasm between your lived experience and the narrative imposed upon you.

This disconnect can lead to a cascade of emotions: anger at being dismissed, fear of future medical encounters, and a deep sense of vulnerability. The very tools designed to aid you — monitors, IVs, surgical instruments — may now evoke anxiety or panic. The sounds of beeping machines can trigger a rush of memories, and the sight of a white coat can send your heart racing.

But it's important to understand that these reactions are valid. They are the echoes of a system that failed to honor your humanity, your autonomy, and your voice. Your trauma is not a result of over-sensitivity; it is a legitimate response to being treated as a case rather than a person.

If I could tell the story of my birth experience without needing to be polite, what would I say?

Let go of making others comfortable. What's your uncensored truth?

> If I could tell the story of my birth experience without needing to be polite, what would I say?

What parts of my memory feel foggy, disjointed, or hard to hold?

Gently note the moments that feel confusing or emotionally "blank." These may be areas where dissociation stepped in to protect you.

What parts of my memory feel foggy, disjointed, or hard to hold?

Where did I feel powerless, overridden, or unseen?

Describe the exact moments when your agency felt dismissed. Your body remembers.

Where did I feel powerless, overridden, or unseen?

What story did others tell me — and how did it conflict with what I lived?

Doctors, nurses, even family may have tried to downplay it. Notice where your inner knowing diverged.

What story did others tell me — and how did it conflict with what I lived?

What do I wish someone had said to me in the aftermath?

Name the words you needed — even if no one offered them.

What do I wish someone had said to me in the aftermath?

If I were to write the medical notes myself, what would I include that they missed?

Give your version.

If I were to write the medical notes myself, what would I include that they missed?

TRACING THE TRUTH

MIRROR REFLECTIONS

Grief can feel invisible because it lives both inside and outside of us. This exercise helps you see your grief from multiple angles.

Why it helps:
Visualizing the difference between inner reality and outer perception makes invisible grief tangible and validates the private experience that others often overlook.

On the inside of the mirror, write what you feel internally — sadness, rage, fear, numbness.
On the outside, write what the world sees (or thinks it sees) — calm, "fine," smiling, coping.

Notice the gap between inside and outside. Reflect on what it feels like to hold both at once.

TRACING THE TRUTH

MIRROR REFLECTIONS

TRACING THE TRUTH

THE GRIEF BOAT

Grief can feel like a heavy weight threatening to pull you under. This exercise gives it a form you can observe, manage, and acknowledge.

Why it helps:
Externalizing grief as a physical object allows you to observe it with compassion and see your capacity to navigate it without being fully submerged.

Label the boat with the grief you are carrying (fear, shame, lost hopes, loss of control).
Around the boat, draw the waves or stormy water that represents triggers or external pressures.
On the shore, write tools, resources, or support that can help steady the boat.

Reflect: Write a reflection. How does the boat move when you engage your support? When do the waves feel overwhelming?

TRACING THE TRUTH

THE GRIEF BOAT

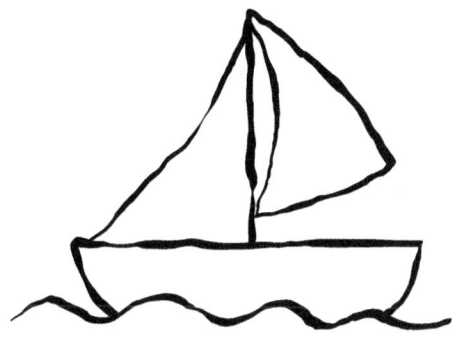

SECTION SEVEN

Invisible Grief – Mourning What Wasn't Supposed to Be Lost

Grief after birth trauma is often invisible. You may not have lost a baby, but you lost something: your safety, your dignity, the experience you imagined, your ability to feel whole in your body, your hope, your trust. And yet... the world often doesn't recognize that loss. People expect you to move on, feel grateful, or celebrate what "went well."

But trauma grief doesn't fit neatly into sympathy cards or baby albums. It's quiet. Lingering. Often silenced — even by ourselves. This section gives you space to say it out loud: I lost something real. And it matters.

You do not need permission to mourn what wasn't supposed to be a loss. You just need space. This is that space — to name it, feel it, and begin the long, slow, sacred process of grieving what was taken, denied, or never got to be. Your heartbreak belongs here.

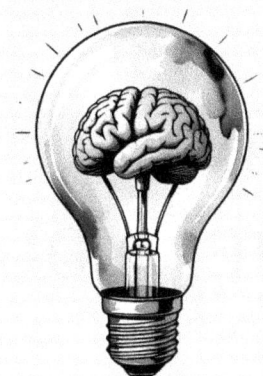

Making Sense Of It
The Grief You Can't See

Grief after birth trauma often slips under the radar. You might not have lost a baby, but the losses are there — profound, real, and persistent. You lost safety in the place where your body was supposed to feel secure. You lost trust in the people who were meant to protect and support you. You lost the birth experience you envisioned, the sense of control over your body, and even the belief that life could be gentle in a moment that demanded vulnerability. These losses don't come with hallmarks or public acknowledgment. They are silent, subtle, and often dismissed, leaving you wondering if they matter — and the answer is yes. Every fragment of what was taken, denied, or distorted matters.

What makes this grief particularly insidious is the gap between internal reality and external expectation. On the outside, life continues. Friends ask, "Isn't the baby healthy?" Partners nod, assuming everything is fine. Healthcare providers may smile, declare "all is well," or fail to see the emotional footprint left behind. But inside, your nervous system is still on alert, your body still storing sensations of overwhelm, and your heart still tethered to the moments that weren't witnessed. This dissonance — between how it feels to you and how the world responds — intensifies isolation. You might question your own reactions, thinking: Am I overreacting? Was it really that bad? Shouldn't I just move on? The answer is simple: no. Your grief is legitimate. Your experience is valid.

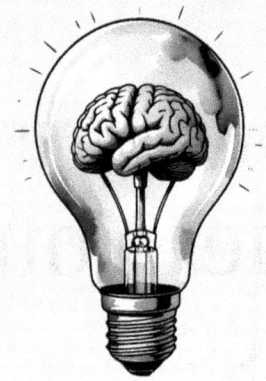

Making Sense Of It
The Grief You Can't See

Culturally, this grief is invisible because society expects birth to be celebratory, linear, and triumphant. The perfect birth story — glowing parents, smiling babies, seamless recovery — leaves no room for the shadow side, the fear, or the rage. Women and birthing people are often told to be grateful, to focus on what "went right," or to simply move on. This societal minimization compounds internal conflict, producing guilt, shame, and self-blame. You are not defective. You are human. You are holding grief that the world has no language for, but which is entirely real.

The first step toward healing is naming your losses, no matter how invisible they seem. When you allow yourself to say, "I lost my sense of safety. I lost my dignity. I lost trust," you begin reclaiming agency over your experience. Witnessing these losses — whether through journaling, speaking with someone who listens, or creating private rituals — is not indulgent; it is essential. It tells your nervous system, your body, and your heart that your grief belongs, that it is valid, and that you will not deny it any longer.

This is also where empowerment begins. By honoring invisible grief, you bridge the gap between what happened and how it is carried. You can start differentiating between the trauma and your identity, between the loss and your worth. Over time, this recognition allows you to navigate life without the weight of unacknowledged sorrow constantly pressing down.

What did I imagine birth would be like — and what did I lose when that wasn't my reality?

Write in detail about the story you hoped for. Give voice to what didn't happen.

What did I imagine birth would be like — and what did I lose when that wasn't my reality?

What part of me feels most broken, left behind, or taken from me?

This may not be a physical loss, but a part of your identity, body trust, or emotional safety.

What part of me feels most broken, left behind, or taken from me?

What grief have I been carrying silently, because it felt "unjustified" or unacknowledged?

Let yourself name it now. No one else needs to validate it for it to be real.

What grief have I been carrying silently, because it felt "unjustified" or unacknowledged?

If someone I loved had gone through what I did, what would I want them to know about their loss?

Sometimes it's easier to find compassion by imagining someone else in our shoes. Then reflect it back inward.

If someone I loved had gone through what I did, what would I want them to know about their loss?

What does my body do when I let myself feel the grief? What happens if I let it soften just a little?

Notice where grief shows up physically — and how gently noticing it shifts your state.

What does my body do when I let myself feel the grief? What happens if I let it soften just a little?

What would a grief ritual look like for me? How might I create space to honor what was lost?

This could be a letter, candle, ceremony, or quiet walk. Grief doesn't always need words — it needs reverence.

What would a grief ritual look like for me? How might I create space to honor what was lost?

SECTION EIGHT

Loving While Still Hurting – Parenting When Bonding Is Hard

No one talks enough about the pain of parenting after birth trauma — especially when bonding doesn't come naturally. You love your child, but you might feel distant. Resentful. Overwhelmed. Or numb. And then comes the guilt: Why can't I just connect? What's wrong with me?

But there's nothing wrong with you. Your nervous system is still trying to feel safe. You're parenting while your body is still recovering from crisis. You're asked to nurture another soul while you're still bleeding emotionally. That's not failure — that's survival.

This section is about compassion. For the version of you who is parenting while hurting. It's about honoring what trauma has interrupted, and gently rebuilding the capacity to connect, little by little, without shame. Bonding is not always instant. Sometimes, love grows through the cracks. And even if no one else sees how hard it is — you are doing something incredibly brave.

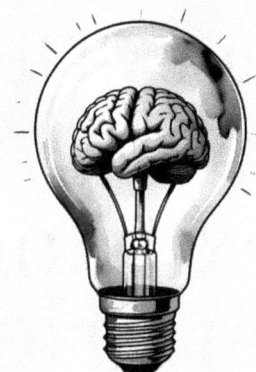

Making Sense Of It
The Complexity of Abortion Grief

Parenting after birth trauma is a paradox. You love your child deeply, yet your body, nervous system, and heart may not feel ready to respond in the ways you imagined. That gap between what you feel and what your body can manage is not a flaw—it's a survival imprint. Trauma rewires the nervous system. During an overwhelming or disempowering birth, the brain prioritizes survival over connection, shifting into protective patterns that may linger for months—or even years. The parts of you meant to relax, attune, and bond may instead remain hypervigilant, watchful, or numb, making acts of closeness like feeding, holding, or playing feel difficult or triggering.

Attachment doesn't vanish because bonding feels delayed. Children are exquisitely responsive not just to consistency of care, but to moments of attuned repair. Even brief, intentional interactions—making eye contact, gentle touch, or calm voice—teach your child that the world is safe, and that they can rely on you. Your nervous system, still recovering, benefits from these small repair cycles too. Trauma-informed research highlights that the act of "showing up imperfectly" repeatedly is more stabilizing than striving for flawless, immediate bonding.

Sociologically, our culture often perpetuates myths of instant parental bonding, portraying love as immediate and unbroken. These expectations deepen shame for parents whose nervous systems are still reeling.

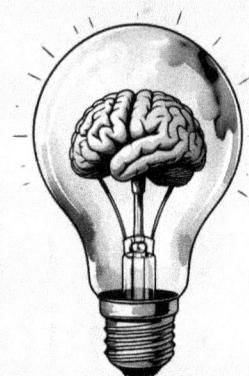

Making Sense Of It
The Complexity of Abortion Grief

Anthropological studies remind us that bonding is rarely immediate across cultures: in many traditional communities, new parents are supported through shared caregiving, ritual, and slow integration into parental roles. In these contexts, gradual attachment is normal, even protective, for both parent and child.

Emotionally, grief, guilt, and shame can intensify feelings of disconnection. Feeling distant doesn't equate to loving less—it reflects the nervous system's ongoing work to feel safe. Compassion—not performance—is the bridge to reconnection. By acknowledging your trauma and granting yourself permission to bond gradually, you cultivate authentic attachment on your own terms.

The process of reconnection is both psychological and somatic. Touch, voice, and rhythm communicate safety to the nervous system. This is why seemingly small, ordinary interactions—holding your child while rocking, humming a song, making eye contact during feeding—become potent acts of co-regulation. You are teaching your system and your child's system simultaneously that closeness is safe.

Your ability to parent through pain is an act of resilience. Healing here is not a timeline; it's a gradual, tender unfolding. Each moment of attunement, even when brief or partial, rebuilds trust, fosters love, and nurtures safety—for both you and your child. You are not failing. You are surviving, repairing, and growing in a way that is deeply human, historically grounded, and biologically sound.

What do I wish I could feel toward my child — and what do I actually feel right now?

Let yourself write without judgment. There is room for both longing and pain here.

What do I wish I could feel toward my child — and what do I actually feel right now?

What messages have I internalized about "what a good parent feels"?

Where did those expectations come from, and how are they helping or hurting me now?

What messages have I internalized about "what a good parent feels"?

When I notice myself emotionally checking out or pulling away, what does that part of me need?

This helps build compassion for the protective patterns — not shame.

When I notice myself emotionally checking out or pulling away, what does that part of me need?

What would I say to a friend who told me they were struggling to bond with their child?

Write it out — then try reading it back to yourself.

What would I say to a friend who told me they were struggling to bond with their child?

What moments (if any) have given me even the tiniest flicker of warmth, love, or presence with my child?

Even a single second counts. Describe it gently.

What moments (if any) have given me even the tiniest flicker of warmth, love, or presence with my child?

What part of me resents the child or the experience of parenting — and can I meet that part with curiosity instead of blame?

This isn't about rejecting the child — it's about exploring your unmet needs.

What part of me resents the child or the experience of parenting — and can I meet that part with curiosity instead of blame?

How does guilt show up in my body? What does my body need when I'm feeling like I'm failing?

Tune in somatically. Explore soothing instead of shaming.

How does guilt show up in my body? What does my body need when I'm feeling like I'm failing?

TRACING THE TRUTH

THE TWO VOICES

Often after trauma, there are two voices inside: one carrying guilt and self-blame, and another carrying truth and compassion. This exercise helps you separate them so you can stop confusing shame with reality.

Why it helps:
By externalizing shame, you weaken its grip and make space for a kinder, more accurate truth. Over time, the compassionate voice becomes easier to access when guilt surfaces.

On the left, write down the painful thoughts that rise when you feel distant from your child (e.g., "I'm failing," "I'm broken," "My baby deserves better").

On the right, respond from the compassionate voice—what a loving friend, therapist, or your future self might say (e.g., "Bonding takes time," "You're surviving something enormous," "Love can grow slowly and still be real").

TRACING THE TRUTH

THE TWO VOICES

Voice of Shame　　　　　　　　　　**Voice of Compassion**

TRACING THE TRUTH

THE THREAD OF CONNECTION

When bonding feels fragile, it can help to notice the smallest threads of connection—those fleeting moments that prove your love is already there, even if it doesn't feel constant. Connection doesn't have to be big, dramatic, or instant. It lives in the little things.

Why it helps:
Your nervous system learns through repetition. By naming and honoring even small moments of attunement, you train your body to recognize that connection is already happening, even if it looks different than you imagined.

Think of one or two small moments where you felt even a flicker of closeness with your child. It might be the way they curled their hand around your finger, the warmth of their body against yours, or the way they looked at you while feeding.
Write them down in vivid detail—what you saw, felt, smelled, or heard.
Next to each one, write: "This is love, too."

TRACING THE TRUTH

THE THREAD OF CONNECTION

ACTION

PROTECTIVE BUBBLE

When emotions run high or interactions feel draining, it's easy for your energy to get scattered. Imagining a soft, light bubble around you helps create a sense of personal space and safety. Using your breath to strengthen the bubble on the inhale and filter in only what feels nourishing on the exhale trains your nervous system to notice boundaries, giving you a calm, centered feeling even in challenging situations.

Sit or stand comfortably, spine tall.

Visualize a soft bubble surrounding your body, glowing lightly.

Inhale and imagine the bubble strengthening, expanding slightly.

Exhale and let in only what nourishes — warmth, safety, or calm.

Continue for 1–3 minutes, noticing a sense of energetic protection and centeredness.

ACTION

SOFT EYES RESET

When we're anxious or hypervigilant, our gaze often narrows, making the world feel tense or threatening. Softening your eyes and expanding your peripheral vision sends a signal to your nervous system that it's safe to relax. This subtle shift can reduce tension in the shoulders, jaw, and chest, helping you feel steadier and more grounded, even in moments of stress.

Sit or stand comfortably with spine tall.

Focus softly ahead, allowing your peripheral vision to widen.

Notice objects to the sides without staring directly at them.

Pay attention to how your body responds — shoulders, jaw, and breath may soften naturally.

Continue for 1–2 minutes, gently returning your focus to soft vision whenever it narrows.

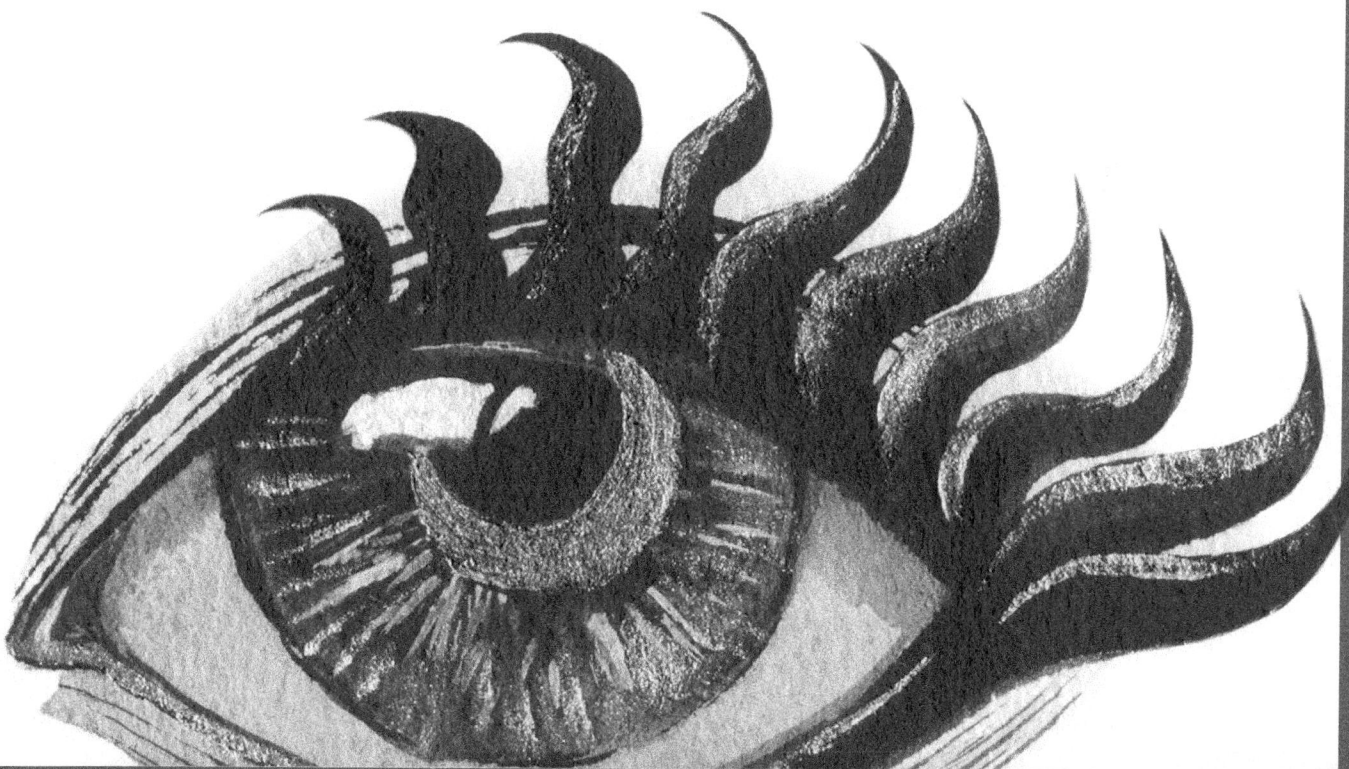

SECTION NINE

If I Ever Do This Again – Fear, Decisions, and Autonomy After Trauma

After surviving birth trauma, the thought of doing it again can feel impossible — or painfully complicated. Some people know they're done. Others grieve the dream of another child they now feel too afraid to try for. Some might consider pregnancy again, but carry a constant undercurrent of dread. And others — perhaps unable to physically carry again — wonder how to process all that's been lost, or what a new path to parenting could look like.

There is no "right" way forward. This chapter is about reclaiming your autonomy. It's about honoring fear without letting it dictate your entire future. Whether you never want to experience birth again, are considering adoption, IVF, surrogacy, or just don't know yet — your experience deserves space, safety, and full permission to evolve.

You've already been through so much. This time, the choice is yours.

Making Sense Of It
Navigating Choice After Trauma

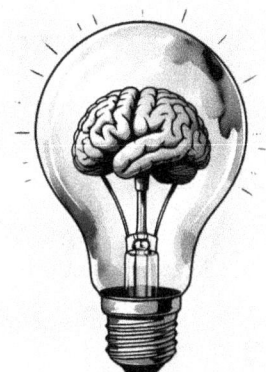

Birth trauma doesn't just imprint on your body or memory—it reshapes your relationship with possibility itself. After surviving something that shook your body, your nervous system, and your sense of agency, the idea of doing it again can feel impossible—or even terrifying. Fear becomes a constant companion, often disguised as rational thinking: "What if it happens again? What if I lose control? What if my body fails me?" These fears are not signs of weakness—they are echoes of survival. Your nervous system remembers what your mind might try to rationalize away, creating a landscape where even imagining a future pregnancy can feel like a tightrope walk above an abyss.

Sociologically, this is amplified by the stories we are told about parenthood. Society frames pregnancy and birth as natural, joyful, and inevitable, rarely acknowledging that trauma fundamentally changes the landscape of possibility. Media, family lore, and casual conversation assume a body that is resilient, a mind unscarred, and desire uniform. When your lived reality doesn't match that narrative, it can feel isolating. Anthropology reminds us that reproductive choices are always embedded in culture, history, and power dynamics. Hesitation, fear, or ambivalence after birth trauma is not an anomaly—it's deeply human and socially understandable. Your body and mind are negotiating a new context: one in which safety, control, and agency have become the center of your experience.

Making Sense Of It
Navigating Choice After Trauma

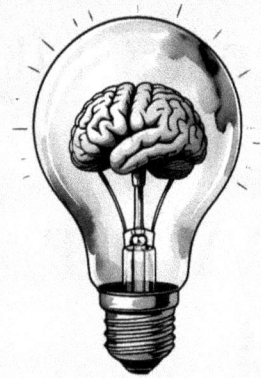

Psychologically, navigating autonomy after trauma is about disentangling fear from choice. Trauma narrows the lens, making "safety first" the default, sometimes at the expense of desire, curiosity, or hope. Healing requires creating space to sit with fear without judgment, to listen deeply to what it tells you about boundaries, limits, and your needs, while weighing it alongside values, dreams, and intuition.

Autonomy is not a single decision—it is a series of micro-decisions, each a reclaiming of your power. Even choosing not to become pregnant, or to pursue alternatives like adoption, surrogacy, or remaining childfree, is an act of agency. You are learning to move from reactive fear toward reflective choice.

Physiologically, trauma leaves a footprint in your nervous system, and reproductive choices trigger that imprint. What feels like hesitation or dread is your body communicating, "I need to feel safe here." Respecting that communication is essential—it is not fear holding you back; it is a map guiding you to make decisions aligned with your well-being. And yet, alongside fear, there can also be hope—tiny, fragile flickers that your future may hold joy and possibility again. Part of reclaiming autonomy is giving yourself permission to feel both: fear and hope, grief and desire, hesitation and curiosity.

If no one else's opinion mattered, what would I want for my future around children or parenting?

Give yourself permission to explore this honestly, without needing a final answer.

If no one else's opinion mattered, what would I want for my future around children or parenting?

What are the fears that come up when I imagine another pregnancy, birth, or child?

Name them. Be specific. Let them breathe.

What are the fears that come up when I imagine another pregnancy, birth, or child?

What losses am I grieving in relation to future children — ones I can't or won't have?

Grief often hides behind fear. Give it room to speak.

What losses am I grieving in relation to future children — ones I can't or won't have?

Are there parts of me that feel I "should" try again? Where does that pressure come from?

Notice if it's internalized messaging, cultural expectation, or someone else's hope.

Are there parts of me that feel I "should" try again? Where does that pressure come from?

What would "reclaiming autonomy" look like for me in this area of my life?

Even if you don't know yet — explore what that phrase stirs in you.

What would "reclaiming autonomy" look like for me in this area of my life?

If I were to try again — through pregnancy, adoption, surrogacy, or otherwise — what would I need to feel safe(r)?

Think emotionally, medically, logistically. Let yourself dream about safety.

If I were to try again — through pregnancy, adoption, surrogacy, or otherwise — what would I need to feel safe(r)?

If I decide not to pursue another child, how can I honor that decision without guilt or apology?

There is strength in knowing your limits and honoring your healing.

If I decide not to pursue another child, how can I honor that decision without guilt or apology?

TRACING THE TRUTH

THE CHOICE GARDEN

Decisions after trauma are like planting seeds. Some grow quickly, some need time, and some may never bloom—and that's okay. This exercise allows you to cultivate your options in a safe, symbolic space.

Why it helps:
Gardening symbolism reinforces that choices don't need to happen all at once. It honors pacing, growth, and care, while giving the reader a visual framework for autonomy, readiness, and self-trust.

Draw a garden on a page with separate plots.
Assign each plot to a possible path (future pregnancy, adoption, surrogacy, staying childfree, etc.).
In each plot, draw the seeds of fear, hope, support, or barriers that affect that choice.

Note what "watering" or "sunlight" each plot needs to grow—these can be self-care, therapy, support networks, medical guidance, or rest.
Reflect: Which plots feel ready to bloom? Which need more time or protection?

TRACING THE TRUTH

THE CHOICE GARDEN

TRACING THE TRUTH

THE CHOICE GARDEN

Reflection:

TRACING THE TRUTH

LETTERS TO YOUR FUTURE SELF

Trauma changes how we approach the future. Writing to your future self allows you to acknowledge fear while gently inviting possibility.

Why it helps:
Letter-writing externalizes internal dialogue, making fear and hope tangible. It strengthens self-compassion and reinforces autonomy by giving your future self permission to evolve without judgment.

Write a letter to yourself 1, 5, or 10 years from now.
Begin by naming your fears: *"I am afraid of…"*
Then speak to your future self with compassion and curiosity: *"I hope that you have…"*
Offer reassurance: *"Whatever you choose, I honor your courage and your right to decide."*

Optional: Keep it sealed, read it later, or destroy it in a ritual that feels safe.

TRACING THE TRUTH

LETTERS TO YOUR FUTURE SELF

TRACING THE TRUTH

LETTERS TO YOUR FUTURE SELF

TRACING THE TRUTH

LETTERS TO YOUR FUTURE SELF

TRACING THE TRUTH

LETTERS TO YOUR FUTURE SELF

TRACING THE TRUTH

THE DECISION RIVER

Choices after trauma often feel like a rushing current—fast, unpredictable, sometimes terrifying. This exercise helps you visualize your options and the emotions that come with them, so you can navigate your river with clarity and compassion.

Why it helps:
Visualizing your choices like a river externalizes fear and hope, letting you see them as coexisting forces rather than opposing enemies. It also gives your nervous system a tangible way to process uncertainty.

Draw a winding river on a blank page.
Label the riverbanks: one side "Fear," the other "Hope."
Place "rocks" in the river for obstacles, doubts, or past trauma triggers.
Place "boats" on the river for each potential choice you're considering (future pregnancy, adoption, surrogacy, staying childfree, etc.).

Note how each boat moves between the banks—does fear hold it back? Does hope push it forward?
Reflect: Which choices feel safest right now? Which feel aligned with your values, even if fear is present?

TRACING THE TRUTH

THE DECISION RIVER

TRACING THE TRUTH

THE DECISION RIVER

Reflection:

ACTION

LEAVES ON A STREAM

We often get stuck in our thoughts, treating them as commands or facts, which fuels stress and emotional overwhelm. Defusion teaches you to step back and see thoughts as just thoughts—mental events that come and go. By visualizing them on leaves drifting down a stream, you give your mind space to notice them without reacting. This practice reduces the pull of negative thinking, strengthens present-moment awareness, and improves emotional flexibility.

Sit quietly and settle. Take a few slow breaths, noticing your body and surroundings.

Visualize the stream. Picture a gentle stream flowing in front of you.

Place thoughts on leaves. Each time a thought appears, imagine putting it on a leaf floating by.

Label hooked moments. If you notice you're caught up in a thought, gently label it "thinking" and return it to the stream.

Continue for 5–10 minutes. Keep observing without judgment, letting each thought drift away.

ACTION

MOMENT-TO-MOMENT AWARENESS

Our minds are constantly busy—hearing, thinking, planning, feeling—and it's easy to get swept away in the stream of thoughts and sensations. This practice helps you step back and notice what's happening in the present without getting stuck. By softly labeling each experience, you create a gentle separation between yourself and the flood of mental activity. Even a short daily practice trains your attention, lowers emotional reactivity, and strengthens the ability to return to calm focus when life gets overwhelming.

Set a timer for 5 minutes so you can fully commit without checking the clock.

Sit comfortably and close your eyes if you like.

Notice experiences as they arise. Softly label them as: "hearing... thinking... planning... feeling..."

Return to your breath. After labeling, bring your attention back to your natural breathing.

Repeat gently. Whenever your mind wanders, notice it, label it, and return to the breath without judgment.

SECTION TEN

The Partner Gap – Feeling Alone in the Aftermath

One of the most painful truths after birth trauma is how isolating it can feel — even with a partner by your side. They may have witnessed the birth, or waited anxiously just outside the door. They may care deeply, but not know how to respond to your pain. They may want to move on, or say, "At least everyone's okay," while you're still waking up in cold sweats, unable to touch your own body.

You're not broken for feeling a gap between what you experienced and how they show up now. Birth trauma often leaves survivors feeling abandoned, dismissed, or emotionally disconnected, even within loving relationships. This section is here to help you name what's been missing, honor your need for understanding, and begin to build (or rebuild) safety — with or without their full comprehension.

Making Sense Of It
Why Trauma Creates a Partner Gap

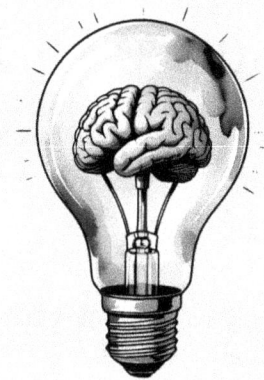

If you survived a birth that broke you, one of the cruellest surprises can be how alone you feel next to the person who shared the room. You both watched the same lights, heard the same beeps — and yet somehow you carry different ghosts. That split is not a moral failing. It's the predictable math of trauma: two people, two nervous systems, two survival stories.

Trauma lodges itself in the body. For the person who birthed, the memory often lives as sensation — the taste of iron, the weight of hands on skin, the sudden, animal-level need to flee or freeze. For partners, the memory is often filtered by helplessness and fear: a corridor of waiting, a pleading voice that couldn't fix things, an image of someone they love becoming small and fragile. Both experiences are real. Both are raw. But they do not line up neatly in time, tone, or shape — and that mismatch becomes the partner gap.

Here are the ways that gap shows up, and what's usually behind it:

- "At least the baby is okay." To a partner, this can be the lifeline they clung to in the moment. To a survivor, it can feel like erasure. Often, this line of reassurance isn't cruelty; it's the partner trying to close a door on terror so they don't collapse under it.

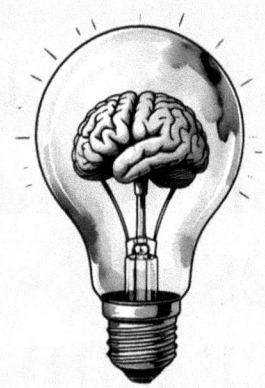
Making Sense Of It
Why Trauma Creates a Partner Gap

- Silence or withdrawal. This looks like absence, but it can also be a defense. Some people shut down to avoid spiraling into panic. Others don't have the language to hold what they saw; staying busy becomes their way to survive.
- Over-functioning, control, or hyper-vigilance. Some partners attempt to "fix" everything after the fact — scheduling appointments, insisting on tests, micromanaging care — because action feels safer than sitting with helplessness.
- Anger, blame, or irritability. Sometimes anger is a stand-in for grief, guilt, or terror — an easier impulse to manage than collapse.

None of this excuses harm. It does, however, explain it. People react to horror with the closest tool they have — and often that tool looks like avoidance, reassurance, busyness, or control. Each of those tools protects a fragile part of them. When those tools collide with your need to be seen, the result is loneliness that cuts deep.

Culturally, this is compounded. Modern childbirth often happens in private, clinical spaces rather than in communal settings where births were witnessed, held, and processed collectively. Anthropologists point out that in many traditional cultures, postpartum care is dense with ritual, presence, and shared labor — an environment that naturally contains shock and grief. In our culture, the couple is left to carry it alone. Partners are expected to be stoic. Mothers are expected to be grateful. There's no script for two people who both hurt in fundamentally different ways.

Making Sense Of It
Why Trauma Creates a Partner Gap

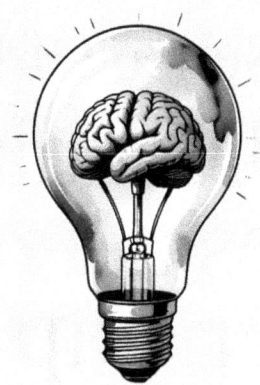

So what does repair look like — in real, practical terms — when one of you is still shaking and the other seems to have moved on?

First: acknowledgment matters more than solutions. Your body wanted a witness in the moment. If your partner didn't — or couldn't — provide one, what helps now is simple and brutal: being seen. Not fixed. Not explained away. Here are practical, concrete things that can help close the gap or at least make it bearable.

Small practices that create real change

- The Witnessing Minute: Set a timer for five minutes. One person speaks without interruption about what they felt; the other listens and then reflects back the emotion (not the fix). Start with: "I felt ___." Listener: "I hear you felt ___." That tiny ritual teaches a partner to hold, not to solve.
- A script for when words fail: If your partner says, "I don't get it," an honest, repair-focused reply could be: "I know you saw hard things too. I don't need you to fix it — I need you to sit with me and say, 'I see you.'" Give them a way to be present that doesn't require psychic perfection.
- Create a 'no-solution zone': Agree on 10–15 minutes where you will not attempt to problem-solve, offer reassurance, or argue logistics. The point is emotional containment, not technicality.
- A short written witness: If talking is too sharp, write. Have each of you write one short paragraph about your moment in the hospital and exchange them. Read aloud. This is often less invasive and lets you hear the person without interruption.
- Micro-requests instead of broad asks: "Sit with me for five minutes and hold my hand" is easier to act on than "Support me." Clear, brief asks lower the bar for participation.

Making Sense Of It
Why Trauma Creates a Partner Gap

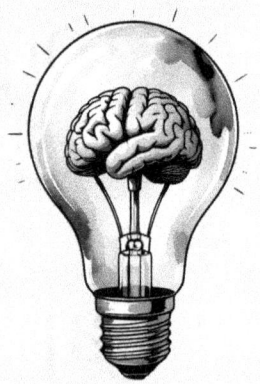

Second: recognize your partner may also be traumatized. They might flinch at hospital smells. They might have nightmares. They might be furious at themselves for not protecting you. That doesn't mean their hurt equals yours; it means both of you need containment. If they won't sit still for sorrow, it may be because their sorrow is a burning thing they're trying not to touch.

Third: you're allowed to protect your healing even from those you love. Wanting distance, needing a boundary, asking for room to process alone — these are valid. Protecting yourself does not make you cruel. It makes you sane.

Fourth: ritual helps where language often fails. There's a reason people throughout history built rites — naming, burning, sewing, burying — to process what the world could not hold. Create a small ritual together: light a candle and name what was hard; or create a "witness box" where you place hospital bands, notes, or photos and open it together months from now. These acts are not sentimental. They are scaffolding for memory and repair.

Finally: recognize when repair isn't possible right now. Sometimes partners cannot meet us — not because they don't love us, but because they are themselves split, terrified, or shut down. That is heartbreak. It is also honest. You can choose to grieve the relationship's limits and still find other carriers: friends, groups, therapists, doulas, community elders. You can ask for a formal witness (a counselor, a mutual friend) to sit with both of you. You can choose to set different expectations for the relationship's emotional labor while you heal.

This is messy. It is unfair. It is real. The partner gap is not proof of failure; it is proof that trauma rewrites how people live together.

What did I need from my partner after the birth that I didn't receive?

Name it without shame. Safety comes from clarity.

What did I need from my partner after the birth that I didn't receive?

How have I felt emotionally alone in this healing process?

You are allowed to tell the truth, even if you love them.

How have I felt emotionally alone in this healing process?

What story does my partner seem to hold about the birth — and how does that differ from mine?

Sometimes pain lives in the silence between two stories.

What story does my partner seem to hold about the birth — and how does that differ from mine?

How have I changed since the trauma, and how have I seen my partner respond to those changes?

Explore both the losses and any surprising strengths.

How have I changed since the trauma, and how have I seen my partner respond to those changes?

What do I wish I could say — without being dismissed, minimized, or interrupted?

Write it like a letter you may or may not send.

What do I wish I could say — without being dismissed, minimized, or interrupted?

Where has my relationship felt safe, and where has it not?

Let yourself feel the full nuance. You can love someone and still feel hurt.

Where has my relationship felt safe, and where has it not?

If I could ask for one specific change or support right now, what would it be?

Get concrete. What would feeling more met look like?

If I could ask for one specific change or support right now, what would it be?

TRACING THE TRUTH

THE LETTER I COULDN'T SAY

So much of the "partner gap" comes from words that never made it out of your mouth — either because the moment passed, they wouldn't have landed, or you just didn't have the strength to speak them. This exercise gives those words a place to live. You don't have to send it. You don't even have to finish it. The act of naming what stayed stuck is healing in itself.

Why it helps:
Unspoken truths become heavy in the body. Writing them down moves them into language, where they can't eat you alive from the inside. Whether you keep, burn, or tear up the letter, the act of writing gives you back your voice.

Let the words come as they are. Write about the silence in the hospital room, the way their eyes avoided yours, the pressure you felt to be "okay" too soon.
If rage comes, write it. If tenderness comes, write that too. You don't need to protect them here. This letter is not about being polite — it's about being honest.
Use prompts to guide you if you get stuck:
"You thought I was okay, but what you didn't see was…"
"When you said __, I needed instead…"
"I wish you could understand that my body still…"
"The silence between us feels like…"
Close your letter with one truth you're ready to hold for yourself:
"Even if you never hear these words, they deserved to be spoken."

TRACING THE TRUTH

THE LETTER I COULDN'T SAY

TRACING THE TRUTH

THE LETTER I COULDN'T SAY

TRACING THE TRUTH

THE LETTER I COULDN'T SAY

TRACING THE TRUTH

THE LETTER I COULDN'T SAY

TRACING THE TRUTH

TWO STORIES, ONE EVENT

One of the hardest parts of birth trauma is realizing you and your partner lived through the same event but walked away with different memories. Instead of trying to force agreement, this exercise helps you hold both truths without erasing your own.

Why it helps:
Seeing the stories side by side helps you externalize the gap, instead of blaming yourself (or them) for it. Both pages can exist without canceling each other out.

Take two sheets of paper. On one, write "My Story." On the other, write "Their Story."
On "My Story," describe what you remember most vividly — the feelings, images, body sensations, and words (or silences) that stayed with you.
On "Their Story," imagine what your partner may have experienced: what they saw, feared, or clung to. Don't censor yourself. This is about perspective, not accuracy.

Place the two pages side by side. Notice the differences. Notice what hurts. Notice what overlaps.

TRACING THE TRUTH

TWO STORIES, ONE EVENT

TRACING THE TRUTH

TWO STORIES, ONE EVENT

TRACING THE TRUTH

TWO STORIES, ONE EVENT

TRACING THE TRUTH

TWO STORIES, ONE EVENT

TRACING THE TRUTH

THE BRIDGE DRAWING

Right now, you may feel a chasm between you and your partner. This exercise lets you visualize that gap, then imagine — even hypothetically — what a bridge might look like.

Why it helps:
Trauma makes the gap feel permanent. Seeing even one possible "plank" creates hope — not by minimizing the distance, but by giving you agency to imagine connection on your terms.

On a blank page, draw two cliffs with space between them. On one side, write your name; on the other, your partner's.
In the space between, write down what makes the gap feel wide: silence, dismissal, different memories, fear, guilt.
Now, sketch or write small planks of a bridge — things that could make connection possible (e.g., listening without fixing, sharing a memory, asking one clear question, saying "I see you").

The bridge doesn't have to be complete. Even one plank is a start.

TRACING THE TRUTH

THE BRIDGE DRAWING

TRACING THE TRUTH

THE BRIDGE DRAWING

ACTION

FEEL IT, DON'T FEED IT

Neuroscience shows that most emotions, if left alone, rise, crest, and fall within about 90 seconds. What keeps us trapped is the story we add — the rumination, replaying, and self-criticism. The 90-Second Emotion Wave helps you move through the raw sensation without getting stuck in the mental loops that amplify pain. By anchoring your attention to your breath and gently offering your body comfort, you allow the emotion to pass through instead of drowning in it. This teaches you that emotions are temporary visitors, not permanent truths.

Set a timer for 90 seconds.

Notice the emotion rise. Imagine it as a wave building. Stay with the body sensations.

Anchor with breath. Breathe slowly, lengthening your exhale. Place a hand where the emotion feels strongest in your body.

Ride the crest. Let the feeling peak without pushing it away or fueling it.

Allow the fall. As the wave settles, ask yourself softly: "What do I need now?"

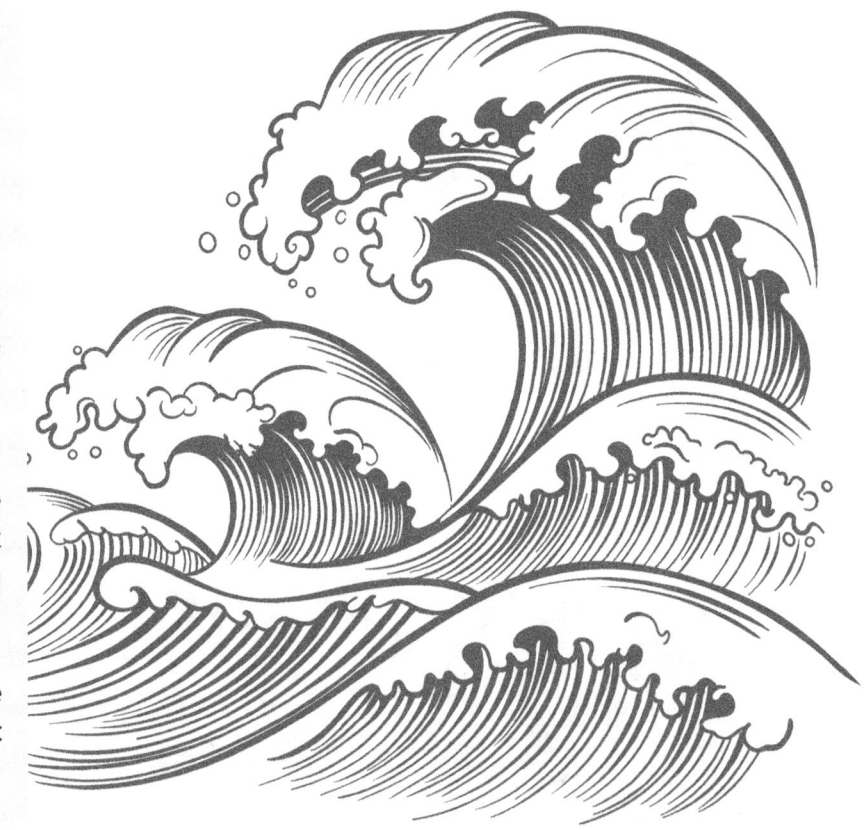

ACTION

KIND INTENTION SETTING

Intentions are like a quiet compass. They don't pressure you or set you up to "succeed" or "fail." They just give you something gentle to return to when the day gets noisy. Starting your morning with one small sentence helps you set the tone: maybe you want to be steadier, softer, braver. Ending the day with another sentence helps you notice where you actually showed up, without the self-punishment. It's less about performance and more about self-trust — proof that you can guide yourself kindly, one day at a time.

Morning: Write one line — "Today, I will show up with ___." (e.g., patience, presence, steadiness).

_____

_____

Carry it lightly: Let it sit in the back of your mind; check in when you feel pulled off course.

Evening: Write one line — "Today, I showed up with ___." Be honest, but kind.

_____

_____

Close the loop: Let the day go. Tomorrow is fresh.

SECTION ELEVEN

When Help Didn't Help – Medical Betrayal and Systemic Gaslighting

You were told to trust the process. Trust the professionals. Trust the system. But instead, what you received may have felt like violation, dismissal, coercion — or complete abandonment. You may have been told everything was "fine" while your body screamed that it wasn't. You may have been minimized when you voiced concern. You may have walked away feeling like your trauma wasn't even acknowledged, let alone validated.

This section is for anyone who has experienced medical betrayal — overt or subtle — during birth. It's also for those still questioning themselves, still wondering if they're "overreacting." You're not. The harm wasn't just physical. It was emotional, psychological, and deeply relational.

When help doesn't help, it hurts more. And the pain of being gaslit by those who were supposed to protect you can ripple for years. This is your space to name it, feel it, and begin to reclaim what was taken — your truth, your voice, your right to bodily autonomy.

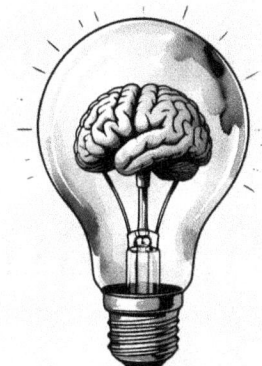

Making Sense Of It
When Help Hurts Instead of Heals

There's the pain of what your body went through. And then there's the pain of what you were told about it. Those are not the same thing — but together, they carve deep scars.

Being gaslit in a medical setting is its own trauma because it's not just neglect; it's erasure. It's standing in a hospital gown, bleeding, terrified, begging with your eyes for someone to see you — and being told, "Everything is fine." It's when the monitor alarms felt louder than your own voice, and yet the people meant to protect you spoke as though nothing alarming was happening. It's when the words "You're overreacting" or "That's normal" crushed your instinct to trust your own body.

This doesn't just hurt in the moment. It fractures something fundamental: your sense that you can rely on others when you're most vulnerable, and that your perception of reality is valid. Trauma is hard enough. But trauma plus betrayal — trauma plus silence — can leave you questioning not just what happened, but who you are for still feeling broken by it.

Here's the truth: when your body screamed and no one listened, you learned something you never should have had to learn — that safety can't be assumed, even in places built for care. That knowledge doesn't just fade. It lingers in the waiting room months later when your chest tightens. It's in the way you Google symptoms instead of calling your doctor, because you've been burned before. It's in the way the phrase "trust the process" now feels like a cruel joke.

Making Sense Of It
When Help Hurts Instead of Heals

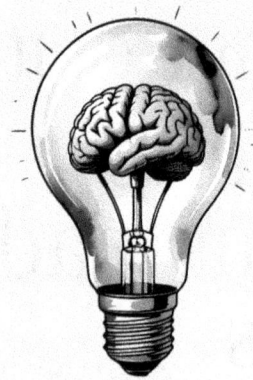

Sociologists would say that institutions are built on trust — we hand over power to doctors and systems because we believe they'll act in our best interest. But when that trust is betrayed, the damage is personal, intimate, and ancestral. Women, in particular, carry generations of stories of not being believed: "She's exaggerating." "She's too emotional." "She's hysterical." Birth trauma often awakens that ancient wound in a very modern form: you spoke, and you weren't heard.

And here's the rawest truth of all: gaslighting is violence dressed up as care. It tells you your body's truth is untrustworthy. It makes you feel crazy for remembering pain that was dismissed. It's why your healing must include this: reclaiming the authority of your own story. Saying, "I was there. I know what I felt. I get to name what was real."

Because until you can stand in that truth, the system keeps winning. And you deserve more than that.

What specific moments during birth or postpartum felt like betrayal to me?

Name them clearly. You're not being dramatic — you're being honest.

What specific moments during birth or postpartum felt like betrayal to me?

What words or actions made me question my own experience?

Gaslighting thrives in silence. You get to break that now.

What words or actions made me question my own experience?

When I think back to the medical professionals involved, what do I feel in my body?

Track sensations: tension, collapse, heat, dissociation. Your body remembers.

When I think back to the medical professionals involved, what do I feel in my body?

What would I have needed instead — in tone, action, or presence — to feel safe?

This isn't fantasy. It's your birthright.

What would I have needed instead — in tone, action, or presence — to feel safe?

Where have I internalized blame that doesn't belong to me?

You do not need to carry their failures as your guilt.

Where have I internalized blame that doesn't belong to me?

If I could speak directly to the person or system that hurt me, what would I say?

Write it like a letter. Don't hold back.

If I could speak directly to the person or system that hurt me, what would I say?

What part of me still doubts my own story — and what does that part need from me?

Bring compassion to the part that's still trying to survive by minimizing.

What part of me still doubts my own story — and what does that part need from me?

TRACING THE TRUTH

REWRITING THE ROOM

Medical gaslighting cuts deep because it leaves you without a witness. No one stepped in to say, "This is not okay." Your body remembers that silence as abandonment. This exercise allows you to create the missing witness you needed in that moment — not to erase what happened, but to bring in the compassion and validation that was absent. By reimagining the scene with someone who finally believes you, you begin to offer your nervous system the repair it deserves.

Why it helps:
By intentionally rewriting the memory with a compassionate figure, you give your body a corrective experience — one where your truth is heard, your pain is validated, and safety is restored. This kind of guided imagery helps reduce the power of the original memory and strengthens your sense of self-trust.

Call up the moment you felt betrayed or dismissed. Notice the details without forcing anything.
Now, imagine a trauma-informed provider entering the room. They meet your eyes, ground the space, and stop the harm.
Hear them say the words your body longed for: "I believe you. What happened was not okay. You matter. You are safe now."
Replay this alternate ending several times until your body feels even a small shift — a breath, a tear, a release of tension.
Write down the exact words your body needed in that moment. Keep them somewhere close, to return to whenever self-doubt creeps in.

TRACING THE TRUTH

REWRITING THE ROOM

TRACING THE TRUTH

REWRITING THE ROOM

TRACING THE TRUTH

REWRITING THE ROOM

TRACING THE TRUTH

REWRITING THE ROOM

ACTION

SEEING THE BIGGER PICTURE

When someone's behavior triggers you—or when you catch yourself blaming yourself—your mind often jumps to the harshest story: "It's all my fault," or "They're deliberately hurting me." Compassionate Reattribution helps you pause and look at the situation more realistically. By considering context, other explanations, and human limits, you can soften blame, see things more fairly, and plan a small step to repair or respond thoughtfully. It doesn't excuse harmful behavior, but it frees your mind from spinning in harsh judgments.

Identify the blamey thought.
Example: "I shouldn't have said that—now they're upset."

Consider other explanations.
Context: maybe they had a rough day.
Skills: maybe they struggle to communicate.
Nervous system: stress can make anyone react sharply.

Choose a fair attribution.
Example: "They were stressed, not necessarily upset at me personally."

Pick one small repair step (if needed).
Example: check in calmly, clarify your intent, or take a pause before responding.

BLAMEY THOUGHT	OTHER EXPLANATIONS	FAIR ATTRIBUTION & REPAIR STEP

ACTION

SEEING THE BIGGER PICTURE

BLAMEY THOUGHT	OTHER EXPLANATIONS	FAIR ATTRIBUTION & REPAIR STEP

ACTION

THE TRIGGER MAP

When you react automatically, it often feels like there's no pause between what happens and how you respond. This exercise helps you slow things down and see the chain of events clearly—what triggered the feeling, the thought that popped up, the urge, and what actually happened. Once you can see it all laid out, you can spot the point where you can intervene next time. That small pause is enough to change the outcome, give yourself more control, and break patterns that have been running on autopilot.

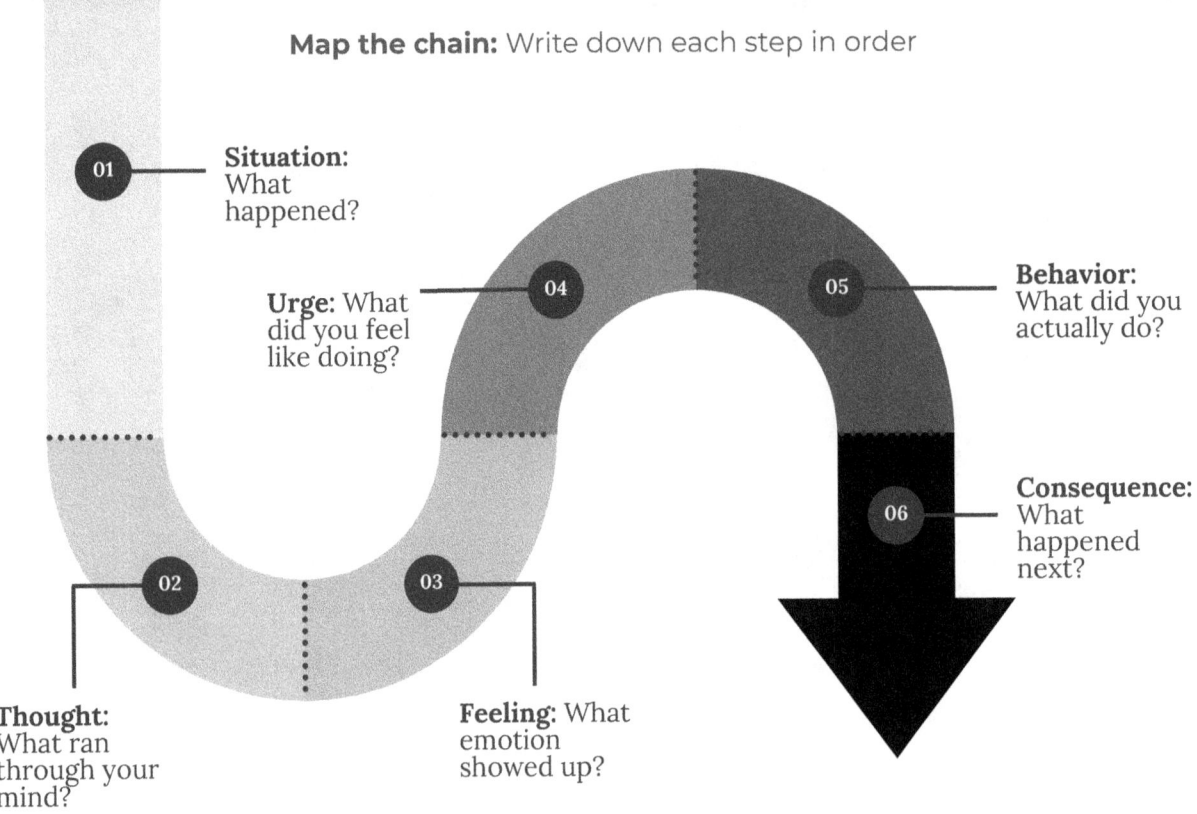

Map the chain: Write down each step in order

01 **Situation:** What happened?

02 **Thought:** What ran through your mind?

03 **Feeling:** What emotion showed up?

04 **Urge:** What did you feel like doing?

05 **Behavior:** What did you actually do?

06 **Consequence:** What happened next?

Circle your change point. Look at the chain and find the first step where you could intervene next time.

Plan one interruption. Pick a tool or skill to use—like a short breathing exercise, a script you can say, or a grounding move—to pause the chain and respond differently.

ACTION

CLIMBING DOWN

When your mind hits you with a brutal thought—like "I always mess up"—it can feel impossible to jump straight to a positive or kind belief. Your brain just won't buy it. This exercise gives you a middle ground. By writing the harsh thought at the top and gradually stepping down to gentler, more realistic versions, you give yourself space to find a statement that actually feels believable. Even if it's not perfect, that 70% believable thought is enough to lower the intensity and guide you toward calmer choices today.

Write the harsh thought at the top rung. (e.g., "I always mess up.")
Step down slowly. Each rung is a slightly softer, more balanced version of the thought.

> "I mess up sometimes, but not always."
> "Everyone makes mistakes. Mine don't erase the things I do well."
> "I can learn from this and try again."

Pick the rung that feels about 70% true. You don't have to land at the bottom. Just stop where it feels believable.
Act from that rung. Let today's choices come from this steadier, more grounded statement.

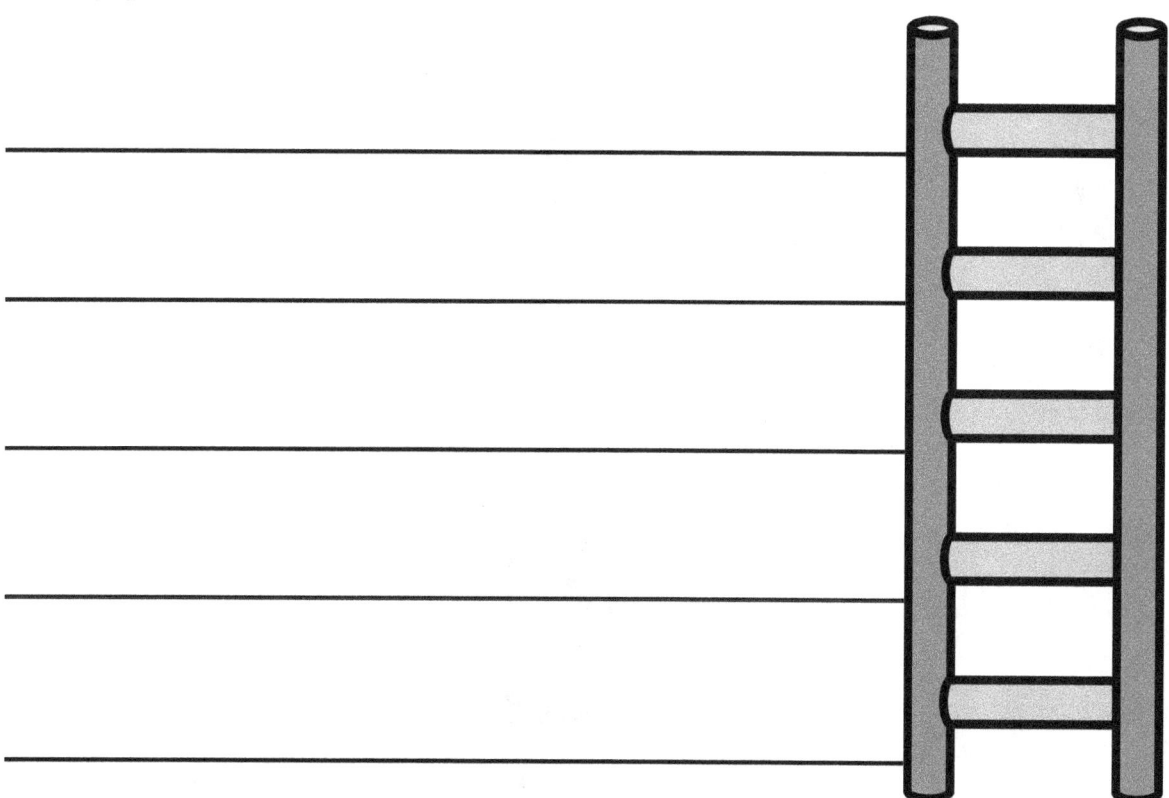

BONUS SECTION

Choosing Safety, Joy, and Permission to Heal

There comes a quiet moment after trauma when the ache begins to loosen — not because the pain is gone, but because something inside you is ready to breathe again. That moment can feel terrifying. Like you're leaving something behind. Like healing means forgetting. Like joy will erase the validity of what you survived.

But healing is not forgetting.

Joy is not betrayal.

Peace is not denial.

This section invites you to practice living again — not by pretending nothing happened, but by letting your nervous system remember what safety, ease, and aliveness can feel like. It's not about bypassing the hard stuff. It's about learning to expand your capacity to hold both pain and pleasure — sorrow and sunlight. You are not broken for wanting to feel good. You're not selfish for reaching for joy. You're allowed to build a life where you can feel safe, free, and connected — even if you're still healing.

Making Sense Of It
Sunlight Through Shadows

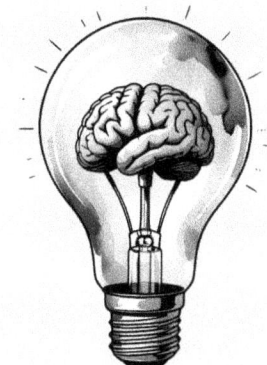

After trauma, the body doesn't immediately believe that danger has passed. Your nervous system, trained to protect you in moments of crisis, can interpret safety as a threat. That's why letting yourself feel joy can feel almost forbidden. Your heart hesitates. Your body tenses. You may feel guilty for laughing, guilty for wanting pleasure, or scared that enjoying life will somehow betray what you endured. This isn't weakness. It's survival.

Grief and trauma do not exist in a vacuum—they unfold inside a social and cultural landscape. Society often sends unspoken rules: "You should be over it by now," "You have a healthy baby, what's the problem?" Anthropology reminds us that trauma is experienced collectively as well as individually. Cultural narratives can invisibilize your pain while simultaneously questioning your right to reclaim joy. Your nervous system remembers the danger even if the world has moved on, creating a tension between inner reality and outer expectation.

Reclaiming safety and joy is an act of radical self-validation. Neuroscience shows that deliberately cultivating moments of safety—through breath, touch, movement, or simple pleasure—helps the nervous system recalibrate. Psychologically, this is about expanding your window of tolerance: learning that you can carry grief and relief, fear and delight, trauma and aliveness, all at once. These micro-moments build resilience and rewrite your internal narrative: that life can feel good, that your body is not broken, and that you deserve pleasure and peace without guilt.

What emotions come up when I imagine feeling better — emotionally, physically, or spiritually?

Does it feel safe? Guilty? Unfamiliar? Let yourself name all of it.

What emotions come up when I imagine feeling better — emotionally, physically, or spiritually?

Have I ever felt afraid of joy, connection, or peace since the trauma?

Describe what happens in your body or thoughts when you feel something good.

Have I ever felt afraid of joy, connection, or peace since the trauma?

If I could define "safety" in my body right now — what would that actually feel like?

Not the idea of safety — the felt sense. Warmth? Spaciousness? Stillness?

If I could define "safety" in my body right now — what would that actually feel like?

What kinds of moments bring me quiet joy or small peace, even now?

List sensory, relational, or spiritual experiences that feel nurturing.

What kinds of moments bring me quiet joy or small peace, even now?

What are some ways I withhold permission from myself to rest, play, or receive support?

Gently explore any internal blocks.

What are some ways I withhold permission from myself to rest, play, or receive support?

If healing didn't mean "getting over it," but "making room for life again" — what would that look like for me?

Visualize your future from that lens.

_____
_____
_____
_____
_____
_____
_____
_____
_____
_____
_____
_____
_____

If healing didn't mean "getting over it," but "making room for life again" — what would that look like for me?

Who am I becoming, now that I am tending to my pain with care instead of fear?

Let this be a celebration — not a pressure to be "healed."

Who am I becoming, now that I am tending to my pain with care instead of fear?

ACTION

SPEAK & STAY STEADY

When emotions run high, it's easy to either go silent or come in too strong. DEAR MAN gives you a clear framework for making requests—or saying no—without guilt or aggression. It balances honesty with effectiveness so you can be heard and respected, even in difficult conversations.

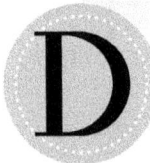

Describe
Briefly state the facts. ("Last week, you didn't follow through on picking up the kids.")

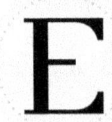

Express
Share how it impacted you. ("I felt really stressed and overwhelmed.")

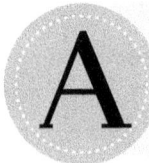

Assert
Clearly ask for what you need. ("I need you to confirm pick-up times in advance.")

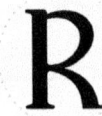

Reinforce
Show the positive outcome. ("That way, we both have more peace of mind.")

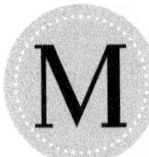

Mindful
Stay on point; don't chase distractions or get pulled into side arguments.

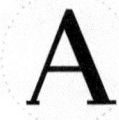

Appear confident
Sit up, steady tone, eye contact if possible. Confidence helps your words land.

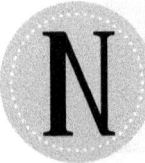

Negotiate
Be flexible; invite collaboration. ("If that time doesn't work, let's pick another together.")

ACTION

CONNECTION FIRST

Relationships often fray not just from big conflicts, but from how we handle the everyday hard moments. GIVE is a simple skill to help you stay connected, even when the conversation is tough. It's about protecting the relationship while still being real. You don't have to agree with someone to treat them with respect—and sometimes, that tone alone changes the entire direction of the exchange.

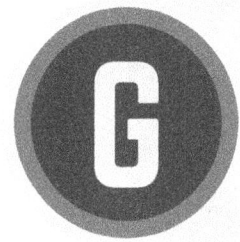

Gentle

No attacks, threats, or judgments. Use a softer start. ("I know this is hard to talk about...")

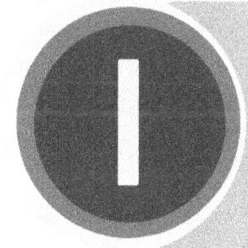

Interested

Really listen. Nod, make space, ask small clarifying questions.

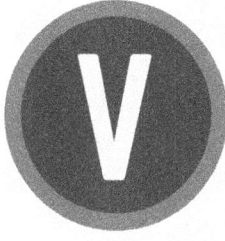

Validate

Acknowledge what makes sense in their perspective, even if you don't agree. ("I see why that would feel stressful for you.")

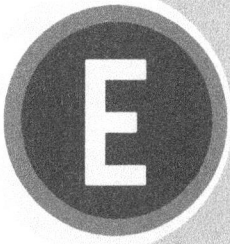

Easy manner

Keep a lightness. Humor if it feels right, relaxed body language, calm tone.

STONEWELL HEALING PRESS

ASSESSMENT

HOW FAR I'VE COME

You've done the work — now let's see where you're at. Take a moment to rate these statements again with honesty and self-compassion. Notice what's shifted, what still feels raw, and what that means for your next steps.

1-10

1. I feel at home in my own body.

2. I can sit with my grief without shutting down.

3. I trust my choices about my body and health.

4. I can experience touch or intimacy without fear.

5. I can speak about my birth experience honestly.

6. I feel emotionally connected to myself and others.

7. I allow myself moments of joy without guilt.

8. I believe my feelings and experiences are valid.

Mindset & Identity Shift Reflection

Healing changes the way you see yourself. You might notice you're less reactive in certain moments, more confident speaking up, or simply softer with yourself. This page is about spotting those shifts — the ones that show you're not the same person who started this journey.

In what ways do I see myself differently than when I started?

What beliefs about myself or others are shifting?

How has my sense of hope, strength, or trust evolved?

MOVING FORWARD

ACTION PLAN

This is your personalized roadmap for continuing growth beyond this workbook. Use this space to clarify which skills you'll keep practicing, how you'll notice early warning signs, and what concrete steps you'll take to support yourself. Remember, transformation happens one intentional step at a time.

Skills I will keep practicing regularly

Early warning signs or triggers I'll watch for:

When I notice these signs, here's what I will do:

MOVING FORWARD

ACTION PLAN

This is your personalized roadmap for continuing growth beyond this workbook. Use this space to clarify which skills you'll keep practicing, how you'll notice early warning signs, and what concrete steps you'll take to support yourself. Remember, transformation happens one intentional step at a time.

Ways I can check in with myself to monitor progress (daily, weekly, monthly):	
People or supports I will reach out to if I need encouragement or accountability:	
One commitment I'm making to myself right now:	

RESOURCE LIST

The resources listed here are shared for informational purposes only. While they provide valuable support and tools for mental health, I am not endorsing or guaranteeing the quality, effectiveness, or availability of their services. It's important to explore these options and verify the details directly on their websites to ensure they align with your personal needs.

National Alliance on Mental Illness

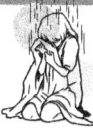

www.nami.org

Offers free mental health education, peer support, and a 24/7 helpline.

Insight Timer

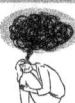

www.insighttimer.com

A free meditation app with thousands of guided meditations, music, and talks on mental well-being

Planned Parenthood

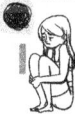

www.plannedparenthood.org/international

Offers resources, training, and advice on how parents can support their child's mental health, including guides and printable resources.

Crisis Text Line

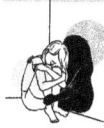

www.crisistextline.org

Offers free, 24/7 text-based support for mental health crises

7 Cups

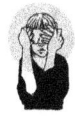

www.7cups.com

Offers free, anonymous online chat with trained volunteers, as well as paid therapy with licensed professionals.

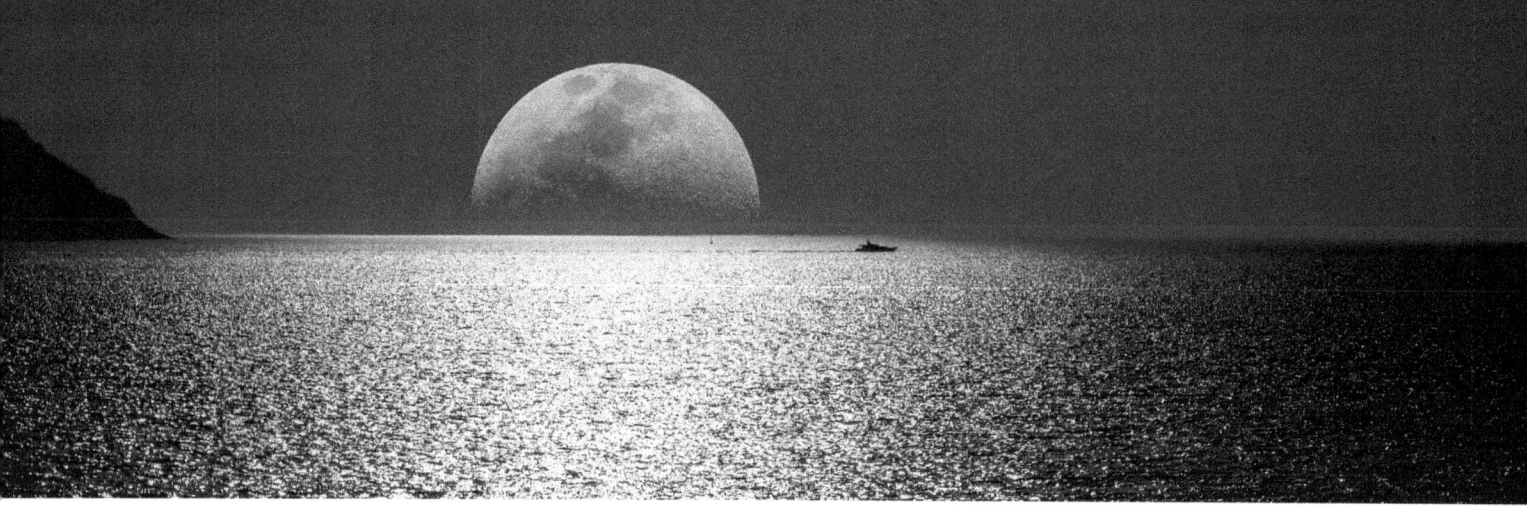

Birth trauma shatters something at the very beginning of what's meant to be one of life's most sacred experiences. You may have walked out of that room with a baby in your arms but a fracture inside you that no one could see. Maybe you felt ignored, violated, dismissed — like your body stopped belonging to you. Maybe you were terrified and no one even noticed. And then, somehow, you were expected to smile. To be grateful. To move on. But trauma doesn't work like that. It lingers. It lives in your muscles, your memories, your parenting, your relationships — sometimes in ways you don't even recognize until years later. And the worst part? Most people don't want to hear about it. They want the happy ending. But you deserve more than silence. You deserve to name what happened. To grieve it. To heal on your own terms. This pain doesn't make you weak. It makes you a survivor of something no one prepared you for. And even if no one held you the way you needed back then — you get to hold yourself now, with truth, care, and the gentleness you always deserved.

You don't have to pretend it didn't hurt just because you survived — I see you, and I know what it cost to make it through.

M. Tourangeau
Stonewell Healing Press

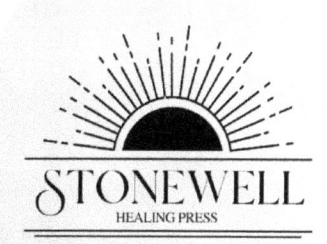

www.ingramcontent.com/pod-product-compliance
Lightning Source LLC
Chambersburg PA
CBHW080411170426
43194CB00015B/2773